T0373232

Interpreter-Mediated Healthcare Communication

Studies in Communication in Organisations and Professions

Series Editor Srikant Sarangi, Aalborg University, Denmark

Founding Editor with Srikant Sarangi: Christopher N. Candlin †

This series aims to build bridges between communication and discourse studies and a broad range of professional, organizational, and workplace sites by foregrounding authoritative analyses of real-life practice – in collaborative, informed and explanatory ways. The series provides an interdisciplinary and interprofessional forum for dialogue between academic researchers and professional/workplace communities and organisations. Examples of appropriate fields of inquiry include: social and community welfare, medicine and healthcare, counselling and therapy, education, law, media, management and business, policy and government and development studies. Coherence among books in the series is achieved through their common concern with cross-over concepts such as power, diversity, identity, agency, decision-making, expertise, risk, appraisal and evaluation.

Published:
Dialogue in Focus Groups: Exploring Socially Shared Knowledge
Ivana Marková, Per Linell, Michele Grossen, Anne Salazar Orvig

Discourse and Responsibility in Professional Settings
Edited by Jan-Ola Östman and Anna Solin

Linguistic Penalties and the Job Interview
Celia Roberts

Understanding and Interaction in Clinical and Educational Settings
Barry Saferstein

Writing the Economy: Activity, Genre and Technology in the World of Banking
Graham Smart

Forthcoming:
Communicative Contingencies in Handling Emergency Medical Calls
Srikant Sarangi

Teamwork and Team Talk: Decision Making across the Boundaries in Health and Social Care
Edited by Srikant Sarangi

Interpreter-Mediated Healthcare Communication

Edited by
Srikant Sarangi

UNIVERSITY OF TORONTO PRESS
Toronto Buffalo London

Reprinted by University of Toronto Press 2024
Toronto Buffalo London
utorontopress.com
Printed and bound by CPI Group (UK) Ltd, Croydon, CR0 4YY

All chapters first published in the journal *Communication & Medicine* Volume 15 Issue 2 (2018)

First published in book form 2024

British Library Cataloguing-in-Publication Data

A catalogue record for this book is available from the British Library.

ISBN-13 978-1-8455-3902-3 (cloth)
978-1-8455-3903-0 (paper)
978-1-8005-0299-4 (PDF)

Library of Congress Cataloging-in-Publication Data

Names: Sarangi, Srikant, 1956- editor.
Title: Interpreter-mediated healthcare communication / edited by Srikant Sarangi.
Description: Sheffield, South Yorkshire ; Bristol, CT : Equinox Publishing Ltd., 2024. | Series: Studies in communication in organisations and professions | "All chapters first published in the journal *Communication & Medicine*, Volume 15, Issue 2 (2018). First published in book form 2024"—title page verso | Includes bibliographical references and index. | Summary: "This book engages - conceptually and empirically - with the ongoing debate concerning the 'influence' occasioned by the participation of an interpreter - whether professionally trained or as a lay family member - in healthcare delivery. Healthcare delivery, especially in the primary care sector, is increasingly becoming multicultural and multilingual in character. This global reality manifests itself as a communicative challenge in interpreter-mediated healthcare consultations, involving professional as well as family members in the role of interpreters. In the context of this book interpreter-mediated healthcare consultations are seen simultaneously as multilingual and multiparty interactions, as well as being dyadic and triadic communication"—Provided by publisher.
Identifiers: LCCN 2022047775 (print) | LCCN 2022047776 (ebook) | ISBN 9781845539023 (hardback) | ISBN 9781845539030 (paperback) | ISBN 9781800502994 (pdf)
Subjects: LCSH: Medicine—Translating. | Health facilities—Translating services. | Communication in medicine.
Classification: LCC R119.5 .I585 2023 (print) | LCC R119.5 (ebook) | DDC 610.1/4—dc23/eng/20221214
LC record available at https://lccn.loc.gov/2022047775
LC ebook record available at https://lccn.loc.gov/2022047776

Typeset by JS Typesetting Ltd, Porthcawl, Mid Glamorgan

Contents

List of Figures and Tables

Figures

Tables

1 Introduction: Communicative vulnerability and its mutation in interpreter-mediated healthcare encounters

Srikant Sarangi

1.1 Introducing interpreter-mediated healthcare encounters

'The field of interpreter-mediated interactions [...] appears to have plateaued in terms of its theoretical development' – so observes Hsieh (2016: 131), in a work in which she endeavours to offer a model of bilingual health communication. Her theoretical model is proposed along the following intersecting parameters at individual and interpersonal levels: communicative goals, individual agency, system norms, quality and equality of care, trust-control-power and temporality. This list of parameters, one could argue, applies to any healthcare interaction – dyadic or triadic – with subtle and not-so-subtle variations observable in interpreter-mediated healthcare communication (IMHC).

A different theoretical angle on IMHC is provided by Greenhalgh *et al.* (2006), drawing explicitly on Habermas's (1984) distinction between 'communicative action' and 'strategic action'. According to Habermas (1990: 63, italics in original):

> Whereas in strategic action one actor seeks to *influence* the behavior of another by means of the threat of sanctions or the prospect of gratifications, in order to *cause* the interaction to continue as the first actor desires, in communicative action one actor seeks to *motivate* another *rationally* by relying on the illocutionary binding/bonding effect (*Bindungseffekt*) of the offer contained in his [sic] speech act.

This distinction between strategic action and communicative action, when applied to IMHC, means that the interpreter seeks to 'influence' rather than 'motivate rationally' the behaviour/understanding of the other participants, i.e. the healthcare provider and the care recipient. Based on empirical data – mainly interviews and focus groups comprising service users and different types of interpreters (professionally trained, family members, allied healthcare professionals/workers) – Greenhalgh *et al.* (2006: 1170) argue that 'the interpreter's presence makes a dyadic interaction into a triad, adding considerable complexity to the social situation and generating operational and technical challenges'. By extension, 'strategic action' from the interpreter in a mediated consultation is unavoidable. This begs the question as to 'how contemporary notions of patient-centredness, shared decision-making, concordance and empowerment might be applied to decision-making in interpreted consultations' (Greenhalgh *et al.* 2006: 1183–1184; Hsieh also makes a similar point when contested goals are imminent).

In extending the theoretical considerations, I see 'communicative vulnerability' constituting the core of the interpreter-mediated healthcare encounter, which is simultaneously multilingual and multiparty in nature. More generally, illness – whether acute or chronic – is a state of vulnerability in biomedical terms, as being ill amounts to disruptions to one's health status and, consequently, dependence on expert and non-expert others. High levels of health literacy as well as individual autonomy can be markers of resilience during a state of vulnerability. When it involves patients who lack equipoise in linguistic and socio-cultural terms in addition to their poorer levels of health literacy, they remain dependent on others to manage their vulnerability at the communicative level, making possible the conditions of strategic action and message manipulation. As I suggest elsewhere:

> In a sense, vulnerability is the other end of the competence spectrum, linguistically and communicatively. The notion of vulnerability also extends to include differences and deficits, especially with regard to unequal levels of health literacy with or without linguistic competencies in class-ridden societies. The communicative vulnerability at the linguistic, interactional level is not something that is only brought along by the participants to a given encounter. It is also the case that the interactional trajectory itself can potentially contribute to the emergence of such vulnerability in an intercultural healthcare setting. (Sarangi 2017: 242)

It is this latter point about interaction-induced vulnerability at the contingent level that concerns the contributors to this volume on IMHC. Interpreter-mediated interaction embraces many different institutional settings such as law, social welfare, health and community care, bureaucracy, the corporate sector, the media and academic and other conferences. These various settings defy a unified set of parameters or generic skills for a professionally trained interpreter to follow in a rule-governed way. The interpreting/mediating activity in the healthcare setting has its own unique interactional (Pöchhacker and Shlesinger 2007) as well as multimodal (Davitti 2019) features, underpinned by differential role expectations concerning the interpreter and the other primary participants.

A typical bilingual clinic consultation involving family members as interpreters (Ebden *et al.* 1988) demonstrates communicative vulnerability at both linguistic and socio-cultural levels. In its extreme form, such vulnerability can cause serious misunderstandings and compromise the quality of patient care. The very co-presence of family members – not necessarily as ratified interpreters but simply as companions in paediatric, geriatric, palliative and genetic consultations – does signal a sense of vulnerability on the part of the patient in need of mediation. Traces of communicative vulnerability can also be noticed in any triadic consultation involving professional interpreters. In both scenarios, the absence of mutual competencies in each other's first language or in a common language as far as the main participants are concerned occasions the mediating role of a third party – the interpreter, whether professional or lay[1] – to minimize the communicative barrier.

The effects of the participation of an interpreter, whether a professional or a lay individual, is an ongoing debate. Based on an extensive review of published literature, Karliner *et al.* (2007) found that for those with interpreting needs, use of professional interpreters is more associated with improved clinical care than the use of lay interpreters, and indeed that the former approaches the quality of care for patients without a language barrier. In contrast, Aranguri *et al.* (2006), based on a detailed sociolinguistic analysis of interpreted consultations, found that needing to use an interpreter resulted in less satisfactory communication, both linguistically (e.g. alterations in content/meaning, reinforcement/validation, repetition) and affectively (e.g. absence of rapport-building small talk). As Elderkin-Thompson *et al.* (2001) point out, in situations where allied healthcare professionals, e.g. nurses, act as interpreters, they are likely to provide information congruent with clinical expectations but not with patients' comments and thus slant the interpretations, reflecting unfavourably on patients and undermining patients' credibility. The challenges and consequences surrounding IMHC are bound to be unique to individual encounters, irrespective of the status of the interpreter.

Primarily, in the healthcare setting, the patient or care recipient with a language barrier is communicatively vulnerable because the preferred language of the care provider misaligns with that of the care recipient. This inevitably means that the care recipient does not have the opportunity to verbalize adequately the presenting symptoms or to communicate directly his/her subjective feelings and emotions to the care provider. However, the care recipient's language deficit is only the tip of the iceberg. There can be other layers of vulnerability, ranging from power asymmetries to epistemological uncertainties to cultural differences surrounding the notion of care (see below).

Communicative vulnerability is not only confined to the care recipient but also engulfs the other participants – the healthcare provider and the interpreter. Given that the healthcare provider lacks the interpreter's bilingual competence, s/he has no means to assess the efficiency and accuracy of the transmitted message through back-translation and thus has to accept the interpreter's rendering of the message based on trust. In this sense, the *care provider* is vulnerable, as s/he is unable to access the subjective feelings and emotions in the patient's preferred language, although it is arguable that even in monolingual settings, patients' subjective, experiential meanings may remain tacit. In Kleinman's (1988: 231–232) characterization of the role of the care provider as 'a mini-ethnographer' in their attempt to place themselves 'in the experience of the patient's illness', the language barrier can heighten the obstacle in the way of 'experiential phenomenology', which 'is the entrée into the world of the sick person.' The patient's subjective experience of illness and its management/coping trajectories do not translate unequivocally through the triadic interpreting process. This feature of vulnerability is heightened if each consultation attended by the same patient involves a different interpreter, marking the absence of continuity of care (but see Hsieh 2016 on tensions relating to patient–interpreter vs. provider–interpreter relationships over time).

The professional interpreter is also vulnerable in the face of complex cognitive demands associated with the interpreting task. In addition, s/he is unlikely to be adequately familiar with the patient's illness trajectory, from both epistemological and experiential standpoints. The contingencies of the immediate encounter in most instances will override the interpreter's prior experiences with similar consultations involving other care recipients. In the multiparty encounter, the interpreter may be compelled or nudged to go beyond their code of practice to intervene much more than they should, thus raising ethical tensions.

Lay interpreters may be more vulnerable than professional interpreters in one sense, but the former have access to mutually shared experiential knowledge that the latter may not have. The vulnerability is particularly salient in the case of child and adult lay interpreters when it comes to terminology, which they may be unfamiliar with in their home language (Green *et al.* 2005). Cohen *et al.* (1999), based on interviews with general practitioners in the UK concerning teenagers and children as interpreters, draw attention to an instance where a teenage son interpreting for his mother confused 'stomach' with 'throat':

> [H]e was saying that her stomach was a problem, but she kept on referring to here (points to throat), I said do you mean the stomach or do you mean the throat, he'd actually got the words wrong, he'd thought that stomach had meant throat. (Cohen *et al.* 1999: 173)

1.2 Six different layers of vulnerability in interpreter-mediated healthcare communication

Here, I identify six different layers of vulnerability that characterizes IMHC in all its complexity.

(1) Professional–client encounters in general – and healthcare encounters in particular – are characterized by knowledge asymmetry, with tacit levels of interpretive procedures and frames that are not easily accessible. The expert care provider does not always explain explicitly the causes and consequences of their actions – say, during history taking or physical examination – which leaves both the interpreter and the care recipient communicatively vulnerable. The patient's lifeworld and culturally sensitive belief systems, which are likely to be shared between the patient and the interpreter, can also operate tacitly, thus putting the care provider in a vulnerable position.

(2) The intercultural dimension means that the interpreted consultation has to remain sensitive to the cross-cultural aspects of health and illness (Helman 1985). Napier *et al.* (2014) attest that efficient healthcare

delivery must be based on an alignment between the biomedical culture and its assumptions on the one hand and the broader culture of values and norms on the other: 'When members of a society lack the capacity for self-reflection – i.e., when people find it difficult to assess their own dysfunctional practices – they become vulnerable to choosing bad meaning over no meaning' (Napier *et al.* 2014: 1634). According to Hsieh (2016: 148):

> As interpreters assist in cross-cultural care, they inevitably need to tread in the boundaries of medicine as they bridge the blurry boundaries of medicine, language, and culture. Despite the provider's claim and power over medical expertise, they face challenges in sharing their control over the process of care and meanings of medicine with interpreters in cross-cultural care.

Schouten and Meeuwesen (2006) suggest that the cultural dimension can be broken down into five components: (1) cultural differences in explanatory models of health and illness, (2) differences in cultural values, (3) cultural differences in patients' preferences for doctor–patient relationships, (4) racism/perceptual biases and (5) linguistic barriers. In the clinical setting, the patient at least has some exposure to the target culture, although the quality of secondary socialization will vary greatly among individual patients. The healthcare professional, in contrast, will very likely have had very little exposure to the patient's cultural beliefs and practices, except in their limited experiences through clinical consultations and perhaps through intercultural training modules which may have presented stereotypes of cultures rather than the lived realities. Here, the interpreter in the role of 'cultural broker' – beyond the translator role – comes to the fore in minimizing the patient's communicative vulnerability.

(3) It is important to keep the cultural barrier distinct from the linguistic, and most specifically paralinguistic, barrier. From an interactional sociolinguistic perspective (Gumperz 1982), communication difficulties may be prevalent at the level of contextualization cues and conversational inferences. Talk in the clinic is not only about presentation of symptoms, but also about presentation of self: because of a lack of linguistic/paralinguistic resources, patients may have difficulties in expressing the nature of symptoms (It-ness) as well as in articulating the affective aspects (I-ness) (Roberts *et al.* 2004). The linguistic/paralinguistic deficit on the patient's part, by extension, puts the interpreter in a vulnerable position as far

as self-understanding is concerned, thus potentially affecting optimal communication with the healthcare provider.

(4) The multiparty character of the encounter, which involves the participation of a professional or lay interpreter, adds another layer of vulnerability in the face of interactional contingencies. According to Georg Simmel (1950), dyadic and multiparty relations are qualitatively different: 'In the dyad, the sociological process remains, in principle, within personal interdependence and does not result in a structure that grows beyond its elements' (Simmel 1950: 126). In triadic and multiparty encounters, the immediate reciprocity that the dyad relies on is constrained; there is a possibility of different dyads forming within the triad, thereby threatening the independence and autonomy of the individual participants and causing them to become subordinated. Although Simmel's remarks are generally about forms and structures of social life (inclusive of the dialectic of freedom and constraint, of autonomy and heteronomy), studies in the IMHC setting would benefit by considering the participation dynamics of triadic consultations more critically (for an overview, see Laidsaar-Powell *et al.* 2013). In the paediatric clinic – which is a default triadic healthcare encounter – Silverman (1987) characterizes the parent as carer in a 'chauffeuring role'. Coupland and Coupland (2000) extend Silverman's characterization to the geriatric clinic and show how sons and daughters can become 'mobilisers' through adopting a less or more powerful role through participation. Also, in relation to triadic geriatric consultations in Taiwan, Tsai (2007) observes that the more companions participate in providing information, the less patients themselves volunteer information or respond to doctor's questions asked prior to the companion's intervention. Even with low-participation companions, patients rarely have a full turn to complete an information unit. In such scenarios, the care provider and the carer assume primary participant status, with the care recipient relegated to a vulnerable third-party status – almost in the role of a bystander.

(5) Following from the above, the nuanced status of the interpreter – whether professional or lay – adds to the complexity of the mediated consultation and, potentially, the communicative vulnerability of all participants. The category of 'lay interpreter' is not homogenous – a spouse vs. a child vs. an adult may position themselves differently. Likewise, the category of 'professional interpreter' is not a unified label, with the possibility of many intervening variables. Among others, Singy and Guex (2005) draw attention to differential – even contrasting – role expectations

concerning the professional interpreter. In the context of interpreting in French-speaking Switzerland based on questionnaires and focus groups, they show that while the interpreters (labelled 'Interpreting Cultural Mediators') perceived themselves as active participants in the consultation and took on broad cultural issues beyond language – to bridge the gap between physicians and patients – this view was not shared by physicians and patients. However, some physicians saw the interpreter as a co-therapist in need of specialized training. As one physician put it:

> To sum up, my mediator is trained, with the linguistic knowledge, the knowledge of therapeutic techniques, knowledge of the institution, but also someone who has been through training with me – that is to say I also require from myself that I should be trained with him. (Singy and Guex 2005: 48)

As already indicated, both lay and professional interpreters may facilitate or inhibit the consultation. Ironically, the interpreter runs the risk of becoming a communicative barrier when he or she is meant to minimize the existing communicative barrier between the care provider and the care recipient. That is, in the process of rendering messages the interpreters may render the care provider and/or the care recipient communicatively vulnerable.

(6) A final layer of vulnerability relates to contemporary western healthcare practices and paradigms such as patient-centeredness, patient autonomy, informed consent, shared decision making, concordance etc., where linguistic, communicative and cultural competencies of the care recipients cannot be taken for granted. The different cultural assumptions surrounding the concept of care can disfranchise the patient in terms of participation in the interaction and decision making within and beyond the clinic encounter.

1.3 Some terminological and analytical considerations

Given the complex layering of vulnerability, the metaphor of *mutation* offers a way of capturing the significant levels of alteration that can potentially occur in IMHC as the interpreter routinely shifts between 'just translating' to 'mediating'. The argument that the role of the interpreter goes beyond being a bilingual dictionary and/or a neutral translator has long been made in interpreting studies (e.g. Wadensjo 1998; Roy 1999;

Davidson 2000, 2002; Angelelli 2004, 2005). In many subsequent studies undertaken from within the language/interaction perspective (e.g. Pöchhacker and Shlesinger 2007; Baraldi and Gavioli 2012), the interpreter is shown as not just a linguistic medium/conduit but as one who mediates the consultation, potentially influencing the communicative processes and also the outcomes.

On the surface, the label *interpreter-mediated healthcare communication* (IMHC) suggests that the interpreter's mediating role is designed to have a beneficial effect on the encounter. Other cognate terms such as participation, coordination, interaction and involvement are useful, but they need to be understood as being both distinctive and interrelated – conceptually and empirically. Goffman's (1974, 1981) distinction between 'sphere of participation', based on production and reception formats within the participant framework, and 'sphere of [focused] interaction' readily comes to mind. He illustrates this distinction in reference to the game of bridge, where a kibitzer (non-player) can participate but not interact – s/he can look at one or more hands and join in during the post-mortem discussion (Goffman 1974: 225). In other words, the kibitzer is mainly an onlooker with a ratified participant status during the game, but once the game is over s/he can interact actively with the other players.

As regards the sphere of participation, the interpreter is positioned for the main part as the mouthpiece of the primary participants – the healthcare provider and the care recipient – whereas in relation to the sphere of interaction s/he can take on the role of spokesperson or author or principal, to use Goffman's (1981) terminology concerning the participant framework. Within the sphere of interaction, for instance, the interpreter can initiate a side activity to gather more information or explain certain phenomena by putting on hold the triadic mode and entering into a dyadic mode. In occasions like this, the interpreter assumes the role of primary participant rather than remaining a secondary participant, thus making a framing/footing shift to the sphere of interaction. If the interpreter is a family member, it is not a simple matter to designate who the primary and secondary participants are in such a complex encounter. With regard to the sphere of interaction, it implies not only active involvement in the communication process through dyadic exchanges but also requires participant-pairs (patient–interpreter and physician–interpreter) to have access to shared knowledge and experience at interpersonal and institutional levels. In sum, the spheres of participation and interaction do become conflated in IMHC.

Typically, while the professional interpreter may claim access to professional and institutional knowledge in order to shift from participation to interaction, the lay interpreter will have access to family-based intersubjective knowledge which would allow for a more active – even aggressive – form of interaction. Interactionally, the lay interpreter can background the patient by answering directly the care provider's questions – thus breaching the ideal four-part sequential structure – or by not transmitting everything that transpires in the consultation, thus altering/mutating the content of turns during the interpretive process. An example would be to change a wh-question (e.g. 'when do you feel the pain?') to a yes/no-question (e.g. 'do you feel pain when you lie down?') as well as deleting key message components, which would constitute a form of recontextualization, or in the Habermasian sense, a form of strategic action.

While translation and mediation as communicative activities have been kept distinct, I would like to suggest that they should also be seen as distinct communicative activities. The literature on interpreting suggests that interpreters are not supposed to mediate (cf. the translation vs. interpretation format). In contrast, the literature on mediation suggests that mediators are not supposed to interpret but facilitate the interaction neutrally. As I see it, interpretation and mediation as communicative activities can be mapped onto a cline of participation, with mediation signalling an increased level of participation/involvement. Participation therefore seems to be a key variable in teasing out interpreting and mediating activities in a given encounter involving professional and lay interpreters, with no or little mediation at one end and with taking over the interaction as a primary participant and relegating one of the other primary participants – usually the patient – to a third party status on the other.

There is extensive literature surrounding the role of the professional interpreter in the healthcare setting. An early typology by Bloom *et al.* (1966) identifies three different interpreter roles: taking over the interview, acting as a tool to facilitate communication and working in partnership with the healthcare provider. Davidson (2000) characterizes the professional interpreter as co-interviewer rather than conveyor of information. Leanza (2007) proposes four professional interpreter role categories: system agent, community agent, integration agent and linguistic agent. According to Greenhalgh *et al.* (2006), the interpreter performs a nuanced set of roles – as interpersonal mediator, system mediator, cultural broker, educator, advocate and link worker. Many others have suggested different typologies using different labels and there is consensus that the role-types are rather porous and that they mutate constantly in relation to the contingencies of a given encounter. The nuanced nature of the professional/lay interpreter's role taking (e.g. translator, cultural broker, mediator, gatekeeper etc.), which to a large extent is tacitly manifest across the participation-interaction continuum, can be appraised more fully through the notion of role-set (Merton 1968; see also Sarangi 2010, 2016) and activity/discourse roles (Halvorsen and Sarangi 2015) *vis-à-vis* participation/involvement.

Interactional tensions are likely to emerge when shifting between the various role categories, targeted differentially for communication support (reproducing speech action, organizing turn taking) and for primary participant status (answering questions, seeking clarification, explaining cultural norms, etc.). The interaction order of multiparty mediated encounters is inherently complex in terms of participation framework and participation status (self-presentation and role performance). All the contributors to this volume address, in different ways, the complexity surrounding the concepts of 'participation' and 'role' and their interactional manifestation.

1.4 The individual contributions

The interpreting/mediating role of the interpreter – whether professional or lay – resembles a scaffold with regard to coordinating and facilitating the triadic encounter. The role taking is subject to many contingent variables – and it is these that the contributions to this volume attempt to unveil. In introducing the contributions and in keeping with the earlier remarks, I reinterpret the core arguments by embedding them in the notion of communicative vulnerability and with particular reference to Goffman's (1974) above-discussed distinction between the sphere of participation and the sphere of interaction. The contributions, however, do not allow for a neat clustering, and there are variables across many axes, including professional vs. lay interpreters, primary vs. tertiary care settings and low- vs. high-stake encounters, not to mention the many different linguistic, ethnic and cultural backgrounds represented. The order in which I introduce the individual contributions is necessarily eclectic.

Role expectations concerning the professional interpreter in both face-to-face and telephone formats in different clinical settings remain the focus of Claudia Angelelli's paper. The complexity of the mediated encounter at times occasions the professional interpreter's going beyond the normative role of 'interpreting' to deliver cross-cultural care, which may be regarded as ethically inappropriate. When the interpreter has a medical background, as in one of the clinics here, s/he takes over the history-taking phase of the encounter, following the nurse practitioner's directive. This serves as an example of the interpreter moving from the sphere of participation to the sphere of interaction to minimize the patient's communicative vulnerability. On other occasions, the interpreter may feel compelled to shift his/her normative role to align with the expectations of the co-participants, which means a sense of vulnerability on the interpreter's part.

Staying with the topic of role shifts and their activity-specific configurations at the interactional level, Galina Bolden compares the professional interpreter's interactional routines in cases of misunderstandings and during the physical examination phase of the consultation (see also Bolden 2000). With regard to misunderstandings, the interpreter would actively initiate and resolve specific repair sequences. During the physical examination phase, the interpreter's participation may be minimal, but his/her bodily actions become salient, complementing the verbal actions. In terms of bodily actions, then, the interpreter enters the sphere of interaction, when the patient can be seen as communicatively more vulnerable. What Bolden characterizes as 'interpreting action in context' is not limited to translation, as the act of interpreting is influenced by the interactional contingencies on the one hand and the ongoing medical activity on the other. The interactional contingencies of the multiparty situation, as in Angelelli's case, can demand that the interpreter's role be either amplified or muted in a given interactional environment.

Claudio Baraldi and Laura Gavioli specifically focus on question-answer sequences in the consultation, as the doctor's designing of questions has to be optimized to enable adequate responses for the management of the patient's present condition. In adopting an active mediating stance, the interpreter instantly recognizes the communicative vulnerability of the patient at the linguistic level (what the authors call 'communicative uncertainty') and simultaneously enters the sphere of interaction for the benefit of the patient's understanding. The extended turn design is aimed at minimizing the apparent communicative uncertainty and potential misunderstanding in an anticipatory manner. Like in Bolden's paper, the interpreter steps outside their translating role and intervenes with a role shift to ensure that medically relevant information is optimally communicated. What we see here is that the triadic interaction gives way to dyadic interaction between the interpreter and the patient in the patient's first language, whereby the doctor as one of the primary participants is relegated to a vulnerable third-party status. The doctor does not normally interrupt the dyadic interaction, which signals a form of collusion.

Cecilia Wadensjo considers the professional interpreter's involvement *vis-à-vis* topic control and mutual trust. She suggests that relational exchange is built upon the idea of the interpreter as conversational partner, with the broader argument framed in relation to co-participants' attitudes towards professional interpreters. Different interpreters show different levels of involvement, thus trading selectively between the spheres of participation and interaction. Such variations will have interactional consequences in terms of topic control and the building of rapport and mutual trust. The emotional aspects, for instance, may not be transmitted on all occasions, and this carries a sense of vulnerability. The analytical distinction between 'relaying by displaying' (representing) and 'relaying by replaying' (re-presenting) becomes useful, while also pointing to how face-work can potentially impact the organization and content of talk. To preserve face and credibility 'displaying' rather than 'replaying' vagueness might be preferred by the interpreter.

Mutual understanding and misunderstanding is the topic underpinning the paper by Sione Twilt, Ludwien Meeuwesen, Jan D. ten Thije and Hans Harmsen. With lay interpreters, the quality of interpreting is at stake, including the increased vulnerability of the patient. In the primary care setting, a lay interpreter may facilitate the communication process through their participation/interaction, but there is also a likelihood that their role taking will instead impede it by introducing misunderstandings. Analytically, the authors draw on the notion of reception format of reporter, recapitulator and responder to characterize the lay interpreter's role shifts during the encounter. While the reporter role keeps the interpreter firmly in the sphere of participation, the responder role amounts to entering the sphere of interaction. The more the lay interpreter moves into the sphere of interaction (i.e. taking on the role of responder) the more one party – usually the patient – is relegated to a third-party status, thus rendering them vulnerable. The authors compare instances of good and poor mutual understanding using external criteria, leading to the triangulation of their findings, i.e. the extent to which different interpreting practices can lead to facilitating or inhibiting understanding. They identify key differences in the role of the lay interpreter with regard to omission of content and undertaking of side-talk activities, which at times can exclude the care provider from the sphere of interaction.

The role of the lay interpreter – as facilitator, as intermediary and as direct source – parallels the position taken by Celia Roberts and Srikant Sarangi, who consider family members as interpreters and more generally as companions in the primary care setting. They compare two settings: a monolingual triadic scenario, which they describe as being a 'mediated consultation', and a bilingual triadic consultation, which they call an 'interpreted consultation'. In the former, the companion/carer in the study plays a mediator role and becomes a ratified co-narrator in expanding and/or streamlining the patient's contributions, while occasionally challenging the patient's account of affairs. Thus the companion/carer moves in and out of the spheres of participation and interaction effortlessly in terms of both activity-specificity and topic-specificity, albeit with different communicative consequences. In the interpreted consultation, in contrast, the lay interpreter does not translate everything for her mother, choosing protection over autonomy. When the patient is unable to participate in the language of the clinic, the carer's interpreting and mediating roles become conflated, requiring the doctor to have 'communicative dexterity'. According to Roberts and Sarangi, lay interpreter-mediated consultations are quite similar to triadic monolingual consultations, which differ in terms of role shifts and alignments from mediated consultations involving professional interpreters. They suggest a cline of mediation as far as lay interpreters/companions are concerned in order to capture the dynamic role alignments in a given encounter.

Charlene Pope and Jason Roberson, based on a comparative study design involving dyadic monolingual and triadic bilingual consultations, examine how shared decision making is accomplished or not in the obstetric clinic – leading to disparity in quality of care. In the triadic consultation, they observe, the normative role expectations may prevent the interpreter from engaging with lifeworld issues, including affective and emotional ones, and humour sequences. As is shown, the sphere of participation and the sphere of interaction unfold differentially in the dyadic monolingual and the triadic bilingual consultations. The findings reveal that, unlike the dyadic monolingual encounter, in the triadic bilingual encounter involving patients with limited English proficiency (LEP) less information is exchanged, as evident in the nature of question-answer sequences – i.e., use of open questions to facilitate participation in the conversational floor vs. closed questions in agenda-specific ways to manage surveillance. Such discrepancies may amount to LEP patients receiving lower-quality care and therefore being vulnerable. More specifically, the nature of shared decision making is rated following an established scale and differences are identified, particularly affecting the LEP patients because of their ethnolinguistic identity.

The paper by Louisa Willoughby, Marisa Cordella, Simon Musgrave and Julie Bradshaw considers a scenario where the healthcare provider is bilingual and uses the patient's first language (Italian) for the consultation, with the bilingual daughter co-present as companion and interpreter. They refer to this scenario as an example of triadic monolingual consultations (language concordant consultations), although there are some elements of bilinguality (use of English in a dominantly Italian consultation). All three participants, because of their shared linguistic repertories, albeit to different levels of competencies, can partake in the sphere of interaction. As the consultation progresses the daughter assumes a supportive role and only occasionally challenges her mother's account of affairs. One is expected to consider the presence of the bilingual doctor as an optimal, even ideal, solution to interpreter-mediated consultations; unlike the monolingual doctor in such triadic interpreted consultations, the bilingual doctor seems to manage the family member's participation more effectively in an attempt to minimize communicative vulnerability.

Finally, Peter Roger and Chris Code deal with the speech pathology clinic, in a setting where the mediating role of the professional interpreter extends to an assessor role. According to them, this setting places 'an excessive cognitive burden' on the interpreter and there are 'special challenges' that can make the interpreter communicatively vulnerable. The interpreter is expected to align their role to that of the speech therapist rather than to perform their normative interpreter role. This means a move from the sphere of participation towards the sphere of interaction in their role as co-assessors of people with aphasia. The tensions are amplified when assessing aphasia as the interpreter orients to message content/meaning and the speech pathologist orients to language form. This differential orientation is underpinned by the goal of assessment concerning what constitutes normal/abnormal language abilities. The 'uninterpretable' nature of many of the utterances produced by speakers with aphasia makes the situation even more complex. In a sense, the interpreter is expected to be activity-focused. but here the interpreter lacks form-specific expertise to carry out the joint assessment. We have a mismatched knowledge schemata at the interprofessional level in terms of production and reception formats, with the interpreter placed in a communicatively vulnerable position. Roger and Code identify three frames: the Testing-Translating frame, the Discussion-Description frame and the Cultural-Linguistic frame. Whereas the Testing-Translating frame can be seen as the default frame belonging to the sphere of participation, the other two frames progressively move the interpreter to the sphere of interaction, thus relegating the person with aphasia to a communicatively vulnerable third-party status. The lack of shared understanding between the two professional groups – speech pathologists and trained interpreters – raises serious questions about the efficacy of such mediated encounters targeted at functional goals.

1.5 Conclusion

In the context of interpreter-mediated healthcare communication (IMHC), when triadic encounters mutate into being dyadic – a development sometimes referred to as side activity – one of the primary participants is excluded from the main participation/interaction frame, making him/her communicatively vulnerable. The vulnerable participant becomes almost a bystander and is not even in the sphere of participation, let alone in the sphere of interaction. The role shifts in the case of both lay and professional interpreters – a theme running through the contributions – are also shifts in frames and footings (Goffman 1981), which can be mapped on to the continuum of the sphere of participation at one end and the sphere of interaction at the other. Viewed from the perspective of Goffman's (1981) participation framework and the associated production and reception formats, mutation may affect the interactional equipoise when one party shifts or is made to shift. The complexity of the encounter and the different configurations/mutations of participation are played out at different levels of role taking and shifts between the spheres of participation and interaction.

Communicative vulnerability also extends to the epistemological positioning of the researcher-analyst, who may not be equally competent in the languages of the clinic as well as being outside the experiential trajectories of illness, the family dynamics involved and the institutional and professional orders in play in a given encounter. A key methodological – and, by extension, analytical – issue concerns what does not get translated/interpreted by the interpreter. In some cases, such omissions and at times misinterpretations are only spotted at the time of transcription and/or translation. Such *post hoc* discoveries pose an ethical dilemma for researchers: what would they do with such incidental findings, something that was not part of the main objective of the study? This needs more systematic investigation, given that such practices are likely to be commonplace in triadic healthcare encounters.

In terms of study designs, our knowledge of what is unique about interpreter-mediated communication would be richer if we knew what goes on when the encounter is not mediated by an interpreter or when it is mediated by a family member whose primary role is not as an interpreter but as a companion/carer, and the language of consultation is the same for the patient and the companion/carer. Other comparative study designs can range from encounters involving native and non-native care recipients (Twilt, Meeuwesen, ten Thije and Harmsen) to mediated (bilingual) and non-mediated (monolingual) consultations involving the same healthcare provider (Pope and Roberson) to triadic monolingual and interpreter-mediated bilingual encounters (Roberts and Sarangi) to the possibility of comparing the communicative practices of bilingual and monolingual doctors involving family members as companions/carers (if we were to extend it to the study by Willoughby, Cordella, Musgrave and Bradshaw). In addition to comparative study designs, triangulation of findings on the basis of external criteria for mutual understanding (Twilt, Meeuwesen, ten Thije and Harmsen) and shared decision making (Pope and Roberson) provides a stronger evidential basis to appraise discourse analytical findings.

Although several studies (e.g. Aranguri *et al.* 2006; Dysart-Gale 2007), including the contributions here, suggest that the presence of the interpreter affects the interaction both positively and negatively; and as with medicine, the good that an interpreter's mediation brings must outweigh any potentially harmful side effects.

Note

1 Researchers use different terminology such as 'formal' (trained, professional) vs. 'informal' (*ad hoc*, proxy, family member) to characterize the status of the interpreter. I here use professional interpreter vs. lay interpreter, while acknowledging that such a distinction becomes blurred

within and across given encounters. This volume covers both types of interpreters. The allied healthcare professional as interpreter falls within the professional–lay continuum.

References

Angelelli, Claudia V. (2004) *Revisiting the Interpreter's Role: A Study of Conference, Court, and Medical Interpreters in Canada, Mexico, and the United States*. Amsterdam: John Benjamins. https://doi.org/10.1075/btl.55

Angelelli, Claudia V. (2005) *Medical Interpreting and Cross-Cultural Communication*. Cambridge: Cambridge University Press. https://doi.org/10.1017/CBO9780511486616

Aranguri, Cesar, Brad Davidson and Robert Ramirez (2006) Patterns of communication through interpreters: A detailed sociolinguistic analysis. *Journal of General Internal Medicine* 21 (6): 623–629. https://doi.org/10.1111/j.1525-1497.2006.00451.x

Baraldi, Claudio and Laura Gavioli (eds) (2012) *Coordinating Participation in Dialogue Interpreting*. Amsterdam: John Benjamins. https://doi.org/10.1075/btl.102

Bolden, Galina B. (2000) Toward understanding practices of medical interpreting: Interpreters' involvement in history taking. *Discourse Studies* 2 (4): 387–419. https://doi.org/10.1177/1461445600002004001

Bloom, Mark, Howard Hanson, Gertrude Frires and Vivian South (1966) The use of interpreters in interviewing. *Mental Hygiene* 50 (2): 214–221.

Cohen, Suzanne, Jo Moran-Ellis and Chris Smaje (1999) Children as informal interpreters in GP consultations: Pragmatics and ideology. *Sociology of Health & Illness* 21 (2): 163–186. https://doi.org/10.1111/1467-9566.00148

Coupland, Nikolas and Justine Coupland (2000) Relational frames and pronominal address/reference: The discourse of geriatric medical triads. In Srikant Sarangi and Malcolm Coulthard (eds) *Discourse and Social Life*, 207–229. London: Pearson.

Davidson, Brad (2000) The interpreter as institutional gatekeeper: The socio-linguistic role of interpreters in Spanish-English medical discourse. *Journal of Sociolinguistics* 4 (3): 379–405. https://doi.org/10.1111/1467-9481.00121

Davidson, Brad (2002) A model for the construction of conversational common ground in interpreted discourse. *Journal of Pragmatics* 34 (9): 1273–1300. https://doi.org/10.1016/S0378-2166(02)00025-5

Davitti, Elana (2019) Methodological explorations of interpreter-mediated interaction: Novel insights from multimodal analysis. *Qualitative Research* 19 (1): 7–29. https://doi.org/10.1177/1468794118761492

Dysart-Gale, Deborah (2007) Clinicians and medical interpreters: Negotiating culturally appropriate care for patients with limited English ability. *Family and Community Health* 30 (3): 237–246. https://doi.org/10.1097/01.FCH.0000277766.62408.96

Ebden, Philip, Oliver J. Carey, Arvind Bhatt and Brian Harrison (1988) The bilingual consultation. *Lancet* 331 (8581): 347. https://doi.org/10.1016/S0140-6736(88)91133-6

Elderkin-Thompson, Virginia, Roxane Cohen Silver and Howard Waitzkin (2001) When nurses double as interpreters: A study of Spanish-speaking patients in a US primary care setting. *Social Science & Medicine* 52 (9): 1343–1358. https://doi.org/10.1016/S0277-9536(00)00234-3

Goffman, Erving (1974) *Frame Analysis: An Essay on the Organization of Experience*. New York: Harper & Row.

Goffman, Erving (1981) *Forms of Talk*. Philadelphia: University of Pennsylvania Press.

Green, Judith, Caroline Free, Vanita Bhavnani and Tony Newman (2005) Translators and mediators: Bilingual young people's accounts of their interpreting work in health care. *Social Science and Medicine* 60 (9): 2097–2110. https://doi.org/10.1016/j.socscimed.2004.08.067

Greenhalgh, Trisha, Nadia Robb and Graham Scambler (2006) Communicative and strategic action in interpreted consultations in primary healthcare: A Habermasian perspective. *Social Science & Medicine* 63 (5): 1170–1187. https://doi.org/10.1016/j.socscimed.2006.03.033

Gumperz, John J. (1982) *Discourse Strategies*. Cambridge: Cambridge University Press. https://doi.org/10.1017/CBO9780511611834

Habermas, Jürgen (1984) *The Theory of Communicative Action, Volume 1: Reason and the Rationalization of Society*. Cambridge: Polity Press.

Habermas, Jürgen (1990) Discourse ethics: Notes on a program of philosophical justification. In Selya Benhabib and Fred Dallmayr (eds) *The Communicative Ethics Controversy*, 60–110. Cambridge, MA: MIT Press.

Halvorsen, Kristin and Srikant Sarangi (2015) Team decision-making in workplace meetings: The interplay of activity roles and discourse roles. *Journal of Pragmatics* 76: 1–14. https://doi.org/10.1016/j.pragma.2014.11.002

Helman, Cecil (1985) *Culture, Health and Illness*. Bristol, UK: Wright.

Hsieh, Elaine (2016) *Bilingual Health Communication: Working with Interpreters in Cross-Cultural Care*. New York: Routledge. https://doi.org/10.4324/9781315658308

Karliner, Leah S., Elizabeth A. Jacobs, Alice Hm Chen and Sunita Mutha (2007) Do professional interpreters improve clinical care for patients with limited English proficiency? A systematic review of literature. *Health Research and Educational Trust* 42 (2): 727–754. https://doi.org/10.1111/j.1475-6773.2006.00629.x

Kleinman, Arthur (1988) *The Illness Narratives: Suffering, Healing, and the Human Condition*. New York: Basic Books.

Laidsaar-Powell, Rebekah, Phyllis Butow, Stella Bu, Cathy Charles, Amiram Gafni, Wendy W. T. Lam, Jesse Jansen, *et al.* (2013) Physician–patient–companion communication and decision-making: A systematic review of triadic medical consultations. *Patient Education & Counseling* 91 (1): 3–13. https://doi.org/10.1016/j.pec.2012.11.007

Leanza, Yvan. (2007) Roles of community interpreters in paediatrics as seen by interpreters, physicians and researchers. In Franz Pöchhacker and Miriam Shlesinger (eds) *Health Interpreting: Discourse and Interaction*, 11–34. Amsterdam: John Benjamins. https://doi.org/10.1075/bct.9.04lea

Merton, Robert K. (1968) *Social Theory and Social Structure* (enlarged edition). New York: Free Press.

Napier, A. David, Beverley Butler, Joseph Calabrese, Angel Chater, Helen Chatterjee, François Guesnet, Robert Horne *et al.* (2014) Culture and health. *Lancet* 9954 (384): 1607–1639. https://doi.org/10.1016/S0140-6736(14)61603-2

Pöchhacker, Franz and Miriam Shlesinger (eds). (2007) *Health Interpreting: Discourse and Interaction*. Amsterdam: John Benjamins. https://doi.org/10.1075/bct.9

Roberts, Celia, Srikant Sarangi and Rebecca Moss (2004) Presentation of self and symptoms in primary care consultations involving patients from non-English speaking backgrounds. *Communication & Medicine* 1 (2): 159–169. https://doi.org/10.1515/come.2004.1.2.159

Roy, Cynthia (1999) *Interpreting as a Discourse Process*. New York: Oxford University Press.

Sarangi, Srikant (2010) Reconfiguring self/identity/status/role: The case of professional role performance in healthcare encounters. *Journal of Applied Linguistics and Professional Practice* 7 (1): 75–95. https://doi.org/10.1558/japl.v7i1.75

Sarangi, Srikant (2016) Activity types, discourse types and role types: interactional hybridity in professional-client encounters. In Donna R. Miller and Paul Bayley (eds) *Hybridity in Systemic Functional Linguistics: Grammar, Text and Discursive Context*, 154–177. Sheffield: Equinox.

Sarangi, Srikant (2017) Mind the gap: 'Communicative vulnerability' and the mediation of linguistic/ cultural diversity in healthcare settings. In Hywel Coleman (ed.) *Multilingualism and Development*, 239–258. London: British Council.

Schouten, Barbara C. and Ludwien Meeuwesen (2006) Cultural differences in medical communication: A review of the literature. *Patient Education & Counselling* 64 (1–3): 21–34. https://doi.org/10.1016/j.pec.2005.11.014

Silverman, David (1987) *Communication and Medical Practice: Social Relations in the Clinic*. London: Sage.

Simmel, Georg (1950) *The Sociology of Georg Simmel*, translated and edited by Kurt H. Wolff. New York: Free Press of Glencoe.

Singy, Pascal and Patrice Guex (2005) The interpreter's role with immigrant patients: Contrasted points of view. *Communication & Medicine* 2 (1): 45–51. https://doi.org/10.1515/come.2005.2.1.45

Tsai, Mei-hui (2007) Who gets to talk?: An interactive framework evaluating companion effects in geriatric triads. *Communication & Medicine* 4 (1): 37–49. https://doi.org/10.1515/CAM.2007.005

Wadensjö, Cecilia (1998) *Interpreting as Interaction*. London: Longman.

Srikant Sarangi was Professor in Humanities and Medicine and Director of the Danish Institute of Humanities and Medicine (DIHM) between 2013 and 2021 at Aalborg University, Denmark, where he continues as Adjunct Professor. Between 1993 and 2013, he was Professor in Language and Communication and Director of the Health Communication Research Centre at Cardiff University, UK, where he continues as Emeritus Professor. In recent years he has been Visiting Professor in many countries, including Finland, Hong Kong, Malaysia, Norway and Qatar. He is author and editor of twelve books, guest editor of ten journal special issues and has published more than 250 journal articles and book chapters in leading journals. Since 1998 he is the editor of *TEXT & TALK: An Interdisciplinary Journal of Language, Discourse and Communication Studies* (formerly *TEXT*) as well as the founding editor, since 2004, of both *Communication & Medicine* and *Journal of Applied Linguistics and Professional Practice* (formerly *Journal of Applied Linguistics*). He is also general editor of the book series *Studies in Communication in Organisations and Professions* (*SCOPE*). Address for correspondence: Department of Communication and Psychology, Aalborg University, Rendsburggade 14, 9000 Aalborg, Denmark. Email: sarangi@ikp.aau.dk

2 Who is talking now? Role expectations and role materializations in interpreter-mediated healthcare encounters

Claudia V. Angelelli

2.1 Introduction

Patients seeking care, providers supplying it and interpreters brokering communication about it may not share expectations about each other's roles, the encounter and the type of knowledge/information transmitted. In addition, co-participants in a healthcare interaction may not share beliefs and practices related to health, diseases, the body, life or mortality. When they come together for a healthcare consultation, a new and cross-cultural community emerges through communication. One may think that responsibilities and roles in this newly formed community mirror those found in a healthcare encounter in which only two interlocutors take part.

This paper investigates the roles and responsibilities in the co-construction of (mis)understanding among patients, healthcare providers and interpreters (Angelelli 2014). Specifically, it aims to shed light on the issues that arise when providers share control of the medical consultation with the interpreter, causing role shifts and blurring role boundaries. After a brief overview of the research on healthcare interpreter-mediated interactions I present segments of provider/patient interactions that illustrate issues faced by interlocutors who engage in communicating health-related information across languages and cultures. I then discuss issues of roles and responsibilities and their implications.

2.2 Literature review: Interpreter-mediated consultations

The assumption of interpreter's non-intervention in communication (Dysart-Gale 2005) is challenged by examining the participation of interpreters during interactions. Studies show that interpreting is a special case of coordinated interaction (Wadensjö 1998; Baraldi and Gavioli 2012), a discourse process (Roy 2000) in which interpreters are co-participants who share responsibility in the talk (Wadensjö 1995) by exercising their agency as they make decisions in the context of their work (Angelelli 2004b). Research on interpreting from cognitive, linguistic and socio-linguistic perspectives help us understand this complex communicative event (De Bot 2000; Paradis 2000; Roy 2000; Sawyer 2004; Russo 2011). Well-documented studies of interpreters in the hospital (Metzger 1999; Davidson 2001; Angelelli 2004a), in the courtroom (Berk-Seligson 2002; Hale 2004), in educational settings (Roy 2000; Valdés *et al.* 2003), in the police station (Berk-Seligson 2009) and in the immigration office (Wadensjö 1995; Hsieh and Hong 2010; Arias-Murcia and López-Diaz 2013; Pollabauer 2017) show that interpreters interact with the parties for whom they facilitate communication by deploying a variety of strategies as they do their work (Wadensjö 1998: 106–108).

Angelelli (2004a: 79–103) has studied a series of strategies interpreters use while facilitating talk in the healthcare setting. She also explores the social factors (such as age, ethnicity, gender, socio-economic status, race) triggering interpreters' participation which result in higher and lower degrees of 'visibility' (exercise of agency) of the interpreter in interactions (Angelelli 2001, 2004b: 68–82). Examples of this are interpreters perpetuating or brokering power differentials between patients and providers, exploring answers, sliding messages up and down the register scale, bridging cultural gaps, expressing affect as well as content and, in some cases, even replacing monolingual interlocutors (e.g., when the doctor tells the interpreter to explore the patient's pain or engage in medical history taking rather than to interpret). As visibility increases, the interpreter's role becomes highly consequential, as it impacts the quality and quantity of information communicated during an interpreted communicative event (ICE) (Angelelli 2004a: 78). It also impacts the provider–patient relationship.

Research also shows that providers and patients have expectations about the interpreter's role: 'For healthcare providers, the interpreter is the instrument that keeps the patient on track; for the patient the interpreter is a co-conversationalist' (Davidson 1998). In a cross-linguistic medical encounter, healthcare interpreters are responsible for facilitating talk between patients and providers who do not share a language or culture.

The difficulties in constructing reciprocal understanding between patients and providers may become magnified when working with linguistically diverse patients. As we will see in the examples below, responsibilities may not always be assumed, role shifts may occur and sometimes are even requested.

2.3 Data and method

The three ICEs studied here are a subset of a corpus consisting of 392 Spanish/English interpreter-mediated consultations (audio-recorded and transcribed) that were collected at California Hope (CH; all names of organizations and persons are fictitious, to protect the identity of the participants) for an earlier study (Angelelli 2004a). The data were collected in accordance with the tradition of ethnography (Fetterman 1998, 2013), and as the sole researcher I was responsible for this and for interaction with participants during observations and interviews. I gained entry to the site and the confidence of the participants by spending a significant amount of time (nine months) getting acquainted with the site and the participants, shadowing interpreters, meeting providers and patients and building trust. All permissions for data collection and protocols for the protection of human subjects were sought and approved both at the field site and the university I represented.

Ten Spanish/English medical interpreters, together with Spanish-speaking patients (representing female and male, the elderly, adults and youngsters – including children), English-speaking healthcare staff (representing physicians, nurses, lab technicians and diabetic educators, to name just a few) and hospital administrators (managers, receptionists) took part in this study. The interpreters are staff members at CH. To be employed, interpreters have to pass a test of medical vocabulary, memory and interpreting skills designed by the Interpreting Service manager. They work eight-hour shifts and interpret face-to-face and over the telephone.

At CH, patients and providers are used to remote interpreting services. The rule is that interpreters work remotely from their cubicles in the Language Services Unit but providers or patients can request to have face-to-face interpreting through bookings. From the corpus, 97%

of the ICEs are remote. Even though the interpreters were physically present in the hospital (they worked from a trailer on the campus), the high percentage of remote ICEs is the manager's strategy to optimize the use of interpreting. The segments selected for this analysis allow us to explore how control over the information requested/provided during the medical encounter is, or is not, retained by healthcare providers during the interpreted medical encounter. Observing, recording and transcribing these encounters, we may identify behaviors such as giving directives to the interpreter to do or not to do something – e.g. 'ask her about chronic illnesses, diabetes, all that...' – rather than communicating directly with the patient and having the interpreter do his/her job. In this example the unpacking of 'all that' is done by the provider for the interpreter, rather than by the interpreter himself; the questions generated by the provider would be meaningful in his/her exploration of the situation, rather than expecting or relying on the interpreter's educated guess. The segments from the encounters exemplify typical provider/patient interactions during the exploratory phase of a medical encounter (Heritage and Drew 1992; Teas Gill and Maynard 2006) at CH. They also align with other reported studies in medical settings (e.g. Wadensjö 1995; Metzger 1999; Bolden 2000; Davidson 2000; Baraldi and Gavioli 2012; Meyer 2012; Gavioli 2012).

2.4 Data analysis

This section discusses three segments of medical interviews. They are typical of interpreter-mediated encounters at CH (see Appendix for transcription conventions).

Medical history taking (Segment 1)

Segment 1 comes from an interview between an elderly Spanish-speaking female patient (P) of Mexican origin and a middle-aged female Caucasian nurse (N) who are face to face in a cubicle with a speakerphone. They are joined remotely by Vicente (I), a staff interpreter from the Language Services Unit at the hospital. Vicente was born in Peru, but had lived for most of his life in Romania, where he became a physician, and at the time of the encounter he had been a staff interpreter at CH for15 years. In Excerpt 1, the nurse needs to find out if the patient has any chronic illnesses. She does not ask the question directly to the patient. Instead, she asks the interpreter to find out the information for her. The request does not contain specific information. Vicente agrees to do so. None of the questions asked by Vicente are given to him by the nurse.[1]

Excerpt 1: I = Interpreter; N = Nurse; P = Patient

01 N: Can you ask her about chronic illnesses, diabetes… all that?
02▶ I: Ahá. Señora Mesa, ¿alguna vez dijo el doctor, aunque sea veinte años atrás, aquí o allá, que tenía usted diabetes?
(*Mrs. Mesa, has a doctor ever told you even twenty years ago here or there that you had diabetes?*)
03 P: No.
04▶ I: ¿Que tenía la presión alta?
(*That you had high blood pressure?*)
05 P: No
06▶ I: ¿Que tenía alguna enfermedad al corazón?
(*That you had heart disease?*)
07 P: Noooo
08▶ I: ¿Que era enferma del hígado?, ¿De los riñones? ¿Del estómago?
(*That you suffered from liver problems? Kidney problems? Stomach problems?*)
09 P: No
10▶ I: ¿Alguna vez la operaron, la internaron? ¿Allá o aquí?
(*Have you ever been operated on or hospitalized? Here or there?*)
11 P: Noooo
12▶ I: ¿Nunca ha estado usted enferma?
(*You have never been sick?*)
13 P: Esteeee si estuve enferma pero… es deeee depresión nerviosa, no de otra cosa
(*Well… I was sick but… it was de… nervous depression… I did not suffer from anything*
else)
14▶ I: Okay… y la internaron por la depresión nerviosa?
(*Okay, and were you hospitalized for nervous depression?*)
15 P: Sí…
(*yes*)
16 I: ¿Allá o aquí?
(*Over there or here?*)
17 P: Esteee… emmm… en Azusa…
(*hmmm..in Azusa*)
18 I: ¿en dónde?
(*Where?*)
19 P: Azusa… cerca de Los Angeles
(*In Azusa, near Los Angeles*)

20▶ I: Ya... she is saying that she denies diabetes, denies cardiovascular disease, denies blood pressure, denies eh... problems with her stomach and her liver... she said that she was... denies surgery... she was admitted once eh... close to Los Angeles... ehmm... for depression
21 N: Okay.. but she does not take any medicine now?
22▶ I: Señora ¿está usted tomando alguna medicina estos días?
(*Ma'am, are you taking any medicine these days?*)
23 P: No
24▶ I: ¿Alguna medicina que compró sin receta?
(*Any over-the-counter medicine?*)
25 P: No
26▶ I: ¿Que trajo de allá, que le dio la comadre Juana?
(*that you brought from there, that Comadre Juana gave to you?*)
27 P: No, nada
(*no, nothing*)
28▶ I: Negative... negative
29 N: Okay, all right... sounds just like she has the blues... her lungs are clear, she is breathing fine and her color looks good I'm gonna check her oxygen saturation and then probably send her home with advice and give her the number to call...
30 I: Okay... Señora dice nuestra enfer
[
(*Okay... our nurse says*)
31 N: [I'll be right back
32 I: [mera que le ha escuchado los pulmones y suenan bien...
(*that she has heard your lungs and they are fine...*)
33▶ P: Síiii
(*Yeees*)
34 I: Dice que su color está bien... que... le va a medir el oxígeno de la sangre
(*that your skin color looks fine... that... and that she will measure the oxygen in your blood*)
35▶ P: Okay
36▶ I: Eso no duele... le va a poner una lucecita en uno de sus dedos solamente por un minuto y después la manda a su casa con unas recomendaciones.
(*That doesn't hurt... and she will put a little light in one of your fingers during one minute and then she will send you home with advice*)
37 P: Okay

(Extract taken from Angelelli 2004a: 94–96)

The nurse does not retain control of the encounter when she addresses the interpreter rather than the patient and directs him to ask the patient about chronic illnesses, diabetes and 'all that' (turn 1). Vicente, the interpreter, not the nurse, does the exploration of the medical history. At turn 2 he starts by addressing the patient by her name and asking her to think back to conversations she has had with her physicians over the last 20 years, both in the US or in Mexico. Vicente does not translate the term 'chronic illness' (turn 2) as '*enfermedad crónica*' but gives a couple of examples to the patient, such as diabetes (turn 2) and high blood pressure (turn 4). Then Vicente shifts register and continues to explore chronic illnesses by naming illnesses after organs that may be affected, such as '*enferma del hígado?, ¿De los riñones? ¿Del estómago?*' (liver problems? Kidney problems? Stomach problems?, turn 8). In his exploration, the interpreter inquired about hospitalization and surgery, and he specifically asked if this has taken place in the country or '*allá*', meaning where the patient is coming from or going back to (turns 10 and 16). He also asked about medicine intake, expanding from prescribed medicine to over-the-counter or traditional/folk medicine (turns 24 and 26). We can see the interpreter unpacking the term 'chronic illnesses' and breaking it down into parts for the patient. The one-line question asked by the nurse in turn 1 is answered with a summary of illnesses and hospitalization (turn 20) and then of medicine intake (turn 28).

Interpreters may or may not be familiar with the protocol used by nurses to explore chronic illnesses; or, an interpreter may be a physician in his own country (as Vicente is) and in following this directive from the nurse, he may ask questions that could be similar to or different from the protocol at CH (resulting in unintentional changes to the standard protocol for exploring chronic illnesses); or the interpreter may take an unnecessarily long time, and then report a summary that may not justify the time involved as the nurse is not informed about the details expressed during the many turns in which she did not participate. These potential outcomes have implications and raise the questions: Who is in charge of obtaining the information? Who is responsible for framing the questions to obtain it? Who is responsible for communicating it to the patient?

It would be tempting to hold the interpreter accountable for stepping out of role (turns 2–20, 24 and 26), taking over the interview or accepting a responsibility that he should not have (turns 32–38). A more mindful look and a more critical approach would turn the tables and see the provider as the party who steps out of role (turns 1 and 21) to become a spectator rather than an actor, using the institutional power she holds (Fairclough 2013) to give directives to the interpreter either explicitly (turn 1) or implicitly (turn 21). Another reading would raise the question of which of the two approaches (i.e. exploring or not exploring the geographic displacement (turns 2 and 10) or the alternative medicine intake (turns 24 and 26), would elicit the required information for the case in hand. Regardless of the approach, in the instances discussed, both the interpreter and the provider (not the patient) share responsibility in how they organize the talk (turns 1, 2–20, 21, 22–28 and 29–36).

The explanation of a procedure (Segment 2)

Excerpts 2 and 3 come from a meeting between Ramira (P), a 39-year-old Mexican female who is in her second month of pregnancy, and Ellen, the genetic counselor (N) who is here to inform Ramira about the different tests available for a pregnant woman of her age. Annette (I), the Spanish-English middle-aged female interpreter, is working remotely. She has been at CH for six months and previously worked as court interpreter. The interview has a total of 207 turns and lasts 35 minutes. In Excerpt 2, we join the conversation at turn 21, as Ellen explains to Ramira why she was referred to genetic counseling.[2]

Excerpt 2

21 N: OK. The reason why Ramira was referred to see me ehmmm it's because of her age of 39 years

22 I: El porque que le recomendaron que se viera con
la señorita esa es debido a la edad de usted de 39 años
(*The reason why you were advised to see this lady is that due to your age, 39 years*)

23 P: Sí... así es...
(*yes, that is so*)

24 N: OK. For all women who are 35 years and more, we offer certain genetic testing to see if the baby could have... a problem such as down syndrome or... mongolism...

25 I: Dice para todas las mujeres que sean de 35 años y mayor (sic), que estén embarazas, ofrecemos varios estudios para verificar... si sus hijos... que esté encargando, verdad...
(*She says that for all women who are 35 or older, who are pregnant, we offer several studies to verify... if the children... that you are expecting... right...*)

26 P: Sí
(*yes*)

27 I: puedan tener posibilidades de sufrir de síndrome de Down, o sea de mongolismo y algunos otra... cosas que... suceden por la edad
(*may suffer from Down syndrome, that is mongolism, and some other things that are caused by age*)

28 P: Sí... esteee... precisamente... Ayer el doctor de allá de Monroe... me mandó

a hacerme… a que me sacaran para hacerme el estudio para el mongolismo
(*yes… ehmm… precisely… yesterday the doctor in Gilroy… sent me to… so that they would draw from me to have the study on mongolism done*)

29 I: OK Pero… ¿fue de sangre o de qué m'hijita?
(*OK but… was it a blood test or what kind of test my dear?*)

30 P: De sangre
(*blood*)

31 I: OK She said yesterday her doctor sent her for a blood test for that

32 N: OK. The blood test and this test are two completely different things. The blood test is only what we call a screening test… ah… and it is called the AFP blood test

33 I: Dice, estos estudios son completamente diferentes. Dice el estudio de sangre es un estudio que se llama la prueba fetal de proteína alfa, ¿verdad?… que es para determinar si hay proteínas… niveles de proteínas producidos por el feto en exceso de cierta cantidad
(*She says that these are two completely different studies. She says that the blood test is a study called alpha protein fetus test, right? And it is to determine if there is protein, the level of protein produced by the fetus over a certain amount*)

34 P: S…

35 I: Go ahead

36 N: OK. So, I'm here right now to offer her this amniocentesis test, because this test is accurate. This tells you for sure if the baby could have a chromosome problem or not

37 I: En este momento ella está ofreciéndole el estudio amniosintesis porque es un estudio que le puede decir claramente si su bebé vaya a tener síndrome de Down o no
(*At this time she is offering you an amniocentesis test because it is a study that can clearly tell you if your baby is going to be a Down syndrome or not*)

38 N: So, what I'm gonna do is explain the whole test to both her and her husband… her husband's here… and… then they need to let me know whether or not they'd like to have this test today

39 I: Y lo que ella va a hacer ahora es explicarle a ustedes, a usted y a su esposo, que está también presente, ¿verdad?)
(*And what she is going to do now is explain to you, to you and to your husband, who is also here, right?*)

40 P: Sí[
(*yes*)

41 I: [cómo va este estudio y para qué,… y entonces ustedes pueden decidir si quieren hacer el estudio hoy o si no. ¿Está bien?
(*what this test is about, what is the purpose, so that you can decide if you want to have this test or not. Okay?*)

42 P: Sí, está bien
(*yes, that is fine*)

43 I: Go ahead

Unlike the previous example, in this interaction the provider seems to be responsible for the information offered to the patient. But, as Ramira shares the information she has received previously about these tests (turn 28), the pattern starts to change. Annette does not relay that information to Ellen directly for her to explore further. Instead, she decides to interrupt Ramira and asks for specifics (turn 29). The way in which Annette addresses Ramira ('my dear', turn 29) shifts from interpreter to co-counselor. Ellen regains control of the interview and explains the differences between the blood test and the amniocentesis test (turns 32, 36 and 38). Ellen divides the information into smaller units and checks for comprehension on the part of the patient. This forces Annette, the interpreter, to stay close to Ellen. The counselor continues with the explanation of the amniocentesis test that she started at turn 36 and makes clear it is optional (turn 38). In Excerpt 3 the conversation begins to break down when the needle is mentioned (turn 49).

Excerpt 3

44 N: OK. The way we do this test is first we do an ultrasound so see how many months pregnant you are and to find a safe place to insert the needle
45 I: Primero, la primerita cosa que hacen es un estudio ultrasonido, ¿verdad?[
(*First, the first thing to do is an ultrasound, right?*)
46 P: [Sí
(*yes*)
47 I: [para determinar cuántos meses tiene usted de embarazo[
(*to determine how many months you are into the pregnancy*)
48 P: [Sí[
(yes)
49 I: [y para ver en qué posición es mejor insertarle la aguja
(*and to know exactly the position into which the needle has to be inserted*)
50 N: Now... she's shaking her head... she doesn't need to have the test but I just need to explain it to her
51 I: Dice... usted no tiene necesidad de recibir el estudio... lo que ella sí tiene obligación de explicarle
(*She says... you don't have to have this test done... but she has to explain it to you*)
52 P: Sí
(*yes*)
53 N: OK. When we insert the needle... I... don't know but they are trying to say something... I don't know what that is
54 I: ¿Qué fue?
(*What's that?*)
55 P: Es que lo que pasa es que me está mostrando aquí en una... en un dibujo[

(*What happens is that she is showing to me on one... drawing*)
56 I: [Aja?
57 P: [este... uno que le están metiendo la jeringa al bebé
(*ehmm... it is a drawing where they are inserting the syringe to the baby*)
58 I: No es al bebé... pero parece[... Yo sé cómo dice
(*no, it is not to the baby, but it looks like it, I know what you mean*)
59 P: [O sea... es a la matriz... o sea dónde está él
(*I mean... to the womb... or where the baby is*)
60 I: Sí... es para sacar un poco de líquido que le rodea al bebé
(*yes, it is to get some of the liquid that surrounds the baby*)
61 P: Aja... entonces yo le pregunté al doctor de allá de Monroe... entonces como yo he tenido problemas con los demás embarazos... de que se me caen a los dos meses y medio
(aha, so I asked the doctor from Monroe, that because I have had problems with the other pregnancies, that I lose them after two and a half months)
62 I: [Mhm
[
63 P: [el doctor me dijo... esteee... me dijo que no me conviene que me hicieran este... este estudio...
(*The doctor told me that this study is not convenient for me*)
64 I: Bien, me permite un momentito entonces, señora....momento eh...
(*All right, just a moment ma'am, one moment please*)
You may not want to go any further with this because she has had problem pregnancies, the doctor and she have discussed this particular study. She said that she's been told by the doctor because she has in the past lost pregnancies, that... emmm.... It wasn't a good test that she should have.... It's not something that he would recommend
65 N: OK. She told me that she had three miscarriages, all at about two and a half months, is that right?
66 I: Yes, that's just what she was just saying
67 N: OK. Ever find a cause for those miscarriages?

At turn 50, Ellen tells Annette that Ramira is shaking her head and emphasizes that Ramira does not have to take the test, but she has to be given the information about it. Annette explains this to Ramira, who seems to understand (turns 51 and 52). When Ellen hears '*sí*' (yes, turn 52), she continues discussing the place where the needle can be inserted using a diagram. Ellen turns to the interpreter for help (turn 53) as she notices a disruption in communication. Between turns 54 and 63, the interaction is between the interpreter and the patient. At turn 67, Ellen wants to explore the causes of previous miscarriages and puts Annette in charge from turns 68 to 80. In Excerpt 4, Annette answers at turn 82 and Ellen continues with the explanation required by protocol.

Excerpt 4

81 N: OK. So they haven't done any studies, that's what I just wanted to know
82 I: No, they have not
83 N: OK. I'm just gonna briefly explain this test of the amniocentesis and if they
don't want to have it, that's fine... but
[
84 I: [Excuse me... I know you know your business much better than I [
85 N: [aha
86 I: [but... I think it'll just make her a little bit more uncomfortable
because she has already, as you've noticed shaken her head
[
87 N: [No
[
88 I: [and said she's discussed it with her doctor and really doesn't feel
comfortable talking about it
89 N: Oh... she told you she doesn't want to talk about it
90 I: That's why she keeps shaking her head no... that she doesn't want the
study... she doesn't want to go further
91 N: Ok. She only shook her head NO one time
92 I: Okeyyyy:
93 N: OK? Umm
94 I: I'll ask her if she wants you to discuss it with her
95 N: Please do
96 I: ¿Señora?
(*ma'am?*)
97 P: Sí
(*yes*)
98 I: Usted quiere que ella siga hablando refiriente a ese procedimiento o
prefiere que no?
(*do you want her to continue talking to you about the procedure or would
you rather not?*)
99 P: Pues, ¿el de la jeringa?
(*well, the one with the syringe?*)
100 I: Aja
(*aha*)
101 P: ¿La jeringa en el... estómago?
The syringe into the stomach?)
102 I: Aja
(*aha*)
103 P: esteee pues la verdad... o sea yo les agradezco que me traten de ayudar
pero... este... en este caso... yo no quiero hacerme ese... estudio... o sea...
quiero que me hagan por ejemplo el... el ultrasonido
(*ehmmm well, truly, I mean, I appreciate that they are trying to help me,
but, ehmmm, in this case do not want to have that study done, I mean I
want to have for example the... the ultrasound*)

104 I: Sí
(yes)
105 P: De... eso... sí... pero el estudio este... de las jeringas... no
(of... that... yes... but this study... of the syringes... no)
106 I: Es muy razonable... me permita (sic)?
(it is very reasonable. Would you allow me?
107 P: Sí
(yes)
108 I: She said she'd rather not go into further discussion with the particular surgery involving the needle. She said she is very grateful that you are offering her this assistance
109 N: OK
110 I: She appreciates it.... She said she would like to go ahead with the ultrasound if that will be at all possible)
111 N: (aja)
112 I: (but she really doesn't want to deal with the needle procedure at all
113 N: OK, that's fine. I need her to sign the refusal now... that she doesn't want to have the amniocentesis test...
114 I: Bien, ¿señora? Ella necesita que usted firme una hoja diciendo que no quiere tener ese estudio con la jeringa
(Ok, ma'am? She needs you to sign a piece of paper saying that you don't want to have this study with the syringe)
115 P: Sí, así es
(yes, that is right)
116 I: She said that's fine. She'll sign it.

Unlike the patient in Segment 1 (Section 4.1), Ramira contributes more actively to role shifting. We see Ramira interacting with Annette as her co- conversationalist (turns 54–64). Instead of requesting information from Ellen or expressing her fears of losing her pregnancy to her, Ramira shares with Annette her decision to have the ultrasound and asks Annette to thank the provider for all her help. Annette accepts the role of co-conversationalist (turn 94) and the request to explain Ramira's decision (turn 98) and advocate for Ramira by advising Ellen not to pursue the explanation of the test (turn 108). Annette thus steps out of role. Ellen tries to regain control and communicate directly with Ramira with Annette's help. Instead, Ellen ends up facing an alliance (turns 84–114) constructed between Ramira and Annette.

The use of pain-rating scale (Segment 3)

The following segment comes from an interview between a middle-aged Spanish-speaking female patient (P) of Mexican origin and a middle-aged female Caucasian nurse (N) who are face to face in a cubicle using a speakerphone system. Mario, a male staff interpreter (I) born in Mexico with eight years of experience at CH, interprets remotely. The patient is complaining about pain in her abdominal area, close to the belly button. In Excerpt 5 we join the conversation as the nurse begins to explore, localize and measure her pain.

Excerpt 5

1 P: Ah, poquito arriba del ombligo
(*Uh, a little above the belly button*)
2 I: Okay, y es, ah, a la derecha o a la izquierda?
(*Okay, and it's, uh, to the right or to the left)*
3 P: Es casi de dirección del ombligo
(*It's almost in direction of the belly button)*
4 I: Ajá, para arribita
(*Uh-huh, a little upwards)*
5 P: Sí, arriba
(*Yes, above)*
6 I: Uh, it's above the belly button.
7 N: Okay, nothing below the belly button?
8 I: No
9 N: Okay, okay from a scale one to ten, ten being the worst, is it a ten?
10 I: ¿Señora?
(*Ma'am?*)
11 P: Sí
(Yes)
12 I: ¿En una escala del cero al diez, siendo cero nada de dolor, el diez un dolor que se muere…
(*On a scale from zero to ten, being zero no pain at all, the ten a pain that you almost die from it*)
13 P: Ajá
(*uh-huh)*
14 I: ¿En qué número pondría usted el dolor?
(*In what number would you place your pain?*)
15 P: El dolor nada más, me, me, me pegaba poquito como con nauseas y se…[
(The pain only, I, I, I, had a little like nausea and it)
16 I: [[[Okay, pero ¿más o menos cuánto?]
(Okay, but more less, how much?)
17 P: Ahh, no mucho, era poquito el dolor.
(*Uh, not much, it was a little pain*)
18 I: Pero en una escala del cero al diez, siendo cero nada de dolor y el diez un dolor que se muere, ¿En cuánto pondría usted el dolor?
(*But on a scale from zero to ten, being zero no pain at all and then a pain that you die, where would you place this pain?*)

19 P: Como un ocho yo creo.
(*About and eight I think*)
20 I: She said an eight
21 N: An eight, okay.

Once it is confirmed that the pain is not below the belly button (turns 7–8), the nurse applies the pain scale (turn 9) to assess its intensity. The nurse does not direct the interpreter to broker the pain scale for the patient, and the interpreter does not focus on answering the nurse's initial close question ('is it a ten?'). Instead, the interpreter takes ten turns (turns 12–21) to broker how the scale works and produces a rating of an eight (turn 21). The nurse does not claim her place in the interaction and accepts the rating co-constructed by the interpreter and the patient without questioning how they arrived at a rating instead of an answer to the 'is it a ten?' question. And, as shown in Excerpt 6 immediately following, the pain rating of 'eight' does not hold.

Excerpt 6

22 P: Porque no'mas (sic) era poquito y me [apretaba el estómago
(Because it was just a little and I would press on my stomach)
23 I: [Entonces señora, ¿si es poquito no es mucho verdad?]
(Then ma'am, if it's a little bit is not a lot, right?)
24 P: No, eh, eh, o sea na'mas (sic) me apretaba el estómago y repetía
*(No, uh, uh, I mean I would just press on my stomach and repeat***)*
25 I: ¿Qué repetía? ¿Usted quiere decir eruptaba?
(*What did you repeat? Do you mean you burped?*)
26 P: Ajá
(*Uh-huh*)
27 I: Okay
28 P: Sí,
(*Yes*)
29 I: Pero, o sea, entonces no, ¿es ocho o menos de ocho?
(*But, I mean, then is not, is it eight or less than eight?*)
30 P: No, es menos de ocho porque se me quitaba luego.
(*No, it's less than eight because it would go away afterwards*)
31 I: Okay, ¿Como cuánto más o menos? ¿E.. era poquito?
(*Okay, how much more less? Was it a little?*)
32 P: Sí, era poquii.. (sic)
(*Yes it was liiitl...*)
33 I: ¿Un tres, un cuatro?
(*A three, a four?*)
34 P: Por ahí, sí, sí, porque un ocho no... es mucho

(Somewhere there, yes, yes because an eight, no, that's a lot)
35 I: [Okay, okay, Pat?]
36 N: Yes? Uh-huh
37 I: It's not eight
38 N: Oh!, which one?
39 I: Uh, she says a little bit, uh, it's around three or four
40 N: Oh, okay, mild then
41 I: Yes, uh, she said at, uh, she had a kind of a gasses (sic), um, that when she was applying pressure she was burping.
42 N: Okay.
43 I: And the, the, the symptoms were a relief.
44 N: Okay, you know, uh, she needs to get a thermometer to check her temperature, okay, this is very important.
45 I: Señora [dice] la enfermera que tendría que tener un termómetro para chequearse la temperatura porque es muy importante tenerlo.
(*Ma'am, the nurse says that you should have a thermometer to check your temperature because it's very important to have it.*)
46 P: [Sí], uh-huh
47 N: Okay, because otherwise, you know what I'm thinking is that she might not even need to come in. It sounds like it's the stomach flu to me. Did she have abdominal cramping also?
48 I: ¿Señora tiene como cólicos?
(*Ma'am, do you have cramps?*)
49 P: Mmmm, no
50 N: Okay and she, uh, was not exposed to anybody that had the stomach flu?
51 I: ¿Señora, ha estado cerca de alguna persona que tenga el flu de estómago?
(*Ma'ma, have you been near someone who has the stomach flu?*)
52 P: Sí
(Yes)
53 I: ¿Ha estado?
(*You have?*)
54 P: Sí, es que a mi, a mi cuñada también así le pegó diarrea, así dice que le dolía el estómago.
(Yes, that's because my, my sister in law had diarrhea, she says that her stomach hurt like this)
55 I: Okay, she said yes, uh, her brother in law had the diarrhea, too.
56 N: Okay, is the pain, um, worse when you move, when she moves or when she coughs?
57 I: ¿Señora el dolor se le pone, se le empeora cuando se, cuando se mueve o cuando tose?
(Ma'am does the pain get, does it get worse when you move or when you cough?)
58 P: Ehh, no, casi no toso.
(*Uh, no I don't really cough*)
59 I: No she doesn't

For the last thirteen turns (turns 47–59) the nurse regains control of the conversation, still exploring the pain as the patient moves or coughs. Segment 3 illustrates another pattern of role shifts. Unlike the provider in Segment 1, this provider tries to retain control of the interview by addressing the patient directly (turns 7 and 9) and directing the interpreter to seek an answer (a rating on the pain scale, turn 56). In his search for the answer, Mario does not keep both parties in direct communication (e.g. turns 22–35). Instead, he does the exploring as the main interlocutor by engaging in 39 consecutive turns (turns 10–38) with the patient and reports the rating back (turns 39) to the provider. The provider does not attempt to recover control of turn taking or of information. She accepts the conversational dynamic as set by the interpreter.

2.5 Discussion and conclusion

The data presented depict typical behaviors observed in provider/patient interactions mediated by an interpreter in this particular hospital context. The segments illustrate the fluidity of roles within segments, and even within turns, which result in role shifts. These shifts impact the construction of mutual understanding among interlocutors, the teamwork required in the patient/provider/interpreter effort to achieve goals in a relationship-centered interaction and the parties' constructions of roles.

Consequently, these shifts also raise questions of responsibility and ethics in talk. Interpreters are not solely responsible for role shifts: responsibility in conversation is shared among co-participants (Hill and Irvine 1993, Sarangi 2012; Solin and Östman 2012). The three parties to the conversation take part in turn taking/receiving/assigning/appropriating (Clyne 1996: 91). Control and power are not monolithic constructions. There are no strict rules followed and role shifts occur frequently.

As evident from the segments presented, when providers relinquish control of the interview and ask interpreters to take over, the communicative goals are less predictable than when providers retain control of the medical discussion and guide interpreters in helping them achieve their goals. The same holds true for the patient and the interpreter. When the patient is able and willing to provide information and answers, or can communicate with both interpreters and providers (e.g. his/her non-familiarity with the pain scale) the conversation may be constructed jointly by the three parties and everyone may be aware of who is saying what to whom.

When interpreters do not play roles perceived as belonging to others (e.g. engage in medical history taking on their own, even when requested by a provider, or accept a responsibility that may jeopardize mutual understanding, even when requested by the patient) and they focus on contributing their renditions to the interpreted-communicative event, mutual understanding and co-construction of meaning is protected. It appears that mutual understanding and co-construction can be achieved if every party to the conversation stays within the expected role.

However, role expectations and materializations appear not to always align in interpreter-mediated provider/patient interactions. The findings in this study align with characterizations of interpreters as gatekeepers, co-conversationalists and advocates, among other roles, and with characterizations of providers who differ in how they maintain control of interviews or transfer control to interpreters. Further research in other language combinations or settings is necessary to shed light on the shared responsibility in construction of understanding or misunderstanding during talk caused by role shifts. This research has implications for the education of interpreters and healthcare providers.

Notes

1 The transcript of this interpreter-mediated encounter was previously used to study (1) the role of the interpreter (Angelelli 2004a) and (2) power and solidarity in interpreter-mediated interaction using critical discourse analysis (Angelelli 2011).

2 The transcript of this interpreter-mediated encounter was previously used to analyze distance and closeness between interlocutors in culturally diverse healthcare communication (Angelelli and Geist-Martín 2005).

References

Angelelli, Claudia V. (2001) *Deconstructing the Invisible Interpreter: A Critical Study of the Interpersonal Role of the Interpreter in a Cross-Cultural/ Linguistic Communicative Event*. Unpublished doctoral dissertation, Stanford University, Stanford, CA.

Angelelli, Claudia V. (2004a) *Medical Interpreting and Cross-cultural Communications*. Cambridge: Cambridge University Press.

Angelelli, Claudia V. (2004b) *Re-Visiting the Interpreter's Role*. Amsterdam: John Benjamins.

Angelelli, Claudia V. (2011) 'Can you ask her about chronic illnesses, diabetes and all that?' In C. Alvstad, A. Hild and E. Tiselius (eds) *Methods and Strategies of Process Research Integrative Approaches in Translation Studies*, 231–246. John Benjamins: Amsterdam. https://doi.org/10.1075/btl.94.17ang

Angelelli, Claudia V. (2014) 'Uh… I am not understanding you at all': Constructing (mis)understanding in provider/patient-interpreted medical encounters. In Melanie Metzger (ed.) *Investigations in Healthcare Interpreting*, 1–31. Washington, DC: Gallaudet University Press.

Angelelli, Claudia V. and Patricia Geist-Martin (2005) Enhancing culturally competent health communication: Constructing understanding between providers and culturally diverse patients. In Eileen B. Ray (ed.) *Health Communication in Practice: A Case Study Approach*, 271–284. Mahwah, NJ: Lawrence Erlbaum Associates. https://doi.org/10.4324/9781410612779-27

Arias-Murcia, Saidy E. and Lucero López-Díaz (2013) Cultural brokerage as a form of caring. *Investigación, Educación y Enfermería* 31 (3): 414–420.

Baraldi, Claudio and Laura Gavioli (eds) (2012) *Coordinating Participation in Dialogue Interpreting*. Amsterdam: John Benjamins. https://doi.org/10.1075/btl.102

Berk-Seligson, Susan (2002) *The Bilingual Courtroom: Court Interpreters in the Judicial Process*. Chicago: University of Chicago Press. https://doi.org/10.7208/chicago/9780226923277.001.0001

Berk-Seligson, Susan (2009) *Coerced Confessions: The Discourse of Bilingual Police Interrogations*. Berlin: Mouton de Gruyter / Chicago: University of Chicago Press. https://doi.org/10.1515/9783110213492

Bolden, Galina B. (2000) Toward understanding practices of medical interpreting: Interpreters' involvement in history taking. *Discourse Studies* 2 (4): 387–419. https://doi.org/10.1177/1461445600002004001

Clyne, Michael (1996) *Intercultural Communication at Work: Cultural Values in Discourse*. Cambridge: Cambridge University Press. https://doi.org/10.1017/CBO9780511620799

Davidson, Brad (1998) *Interpreting Medical Dis-course: A Study of Cross-Linguistic Communication in the Hospital Clinic*. Unpublished doctoral dissertation, Stanford University, Stanford, CA.

Davidson, Brad (2000) The interpreter as institutional gatekeeper: The social-linguistic role of interpreters in Spanish-English medical discourse. *Journal of Sociolinguistics* 4 (3): 379–405. https://doi.org/10.1111/1467-9481.00121

Davidson, Brad (2001) Questions in cross-linguistic medical encounters: The role of the hospital interpreter. *Anthropological Quarterly* 74 (4): 170–178. https://doi.org/10.1353/anq.2001.0035

De Bot, Kees (2000) Simultaneous interpreting as language production. In Birgitta E. Dimitrova and Kenneth Hyltenstam (eds) *Language Processing and Simultaneous Interpreting*, 65–89. Amsterdam: John Benjamins. https://doi.org/10.1075/btl.40.06bot

Dysart-Gale, Deborah (2005). Communication models, professionalization, and the work of medical interpreters. *Health Communication* 17 (1): 91–103. https://doi.org/10.1207/s15327027hc1701_6

Fairclough, Norman (2013) *Language and Power*. London: Routledge.

Fetterman, David M. (1998) *Ethnography: Step-by-Step* (2nd edition). Applied Social Research Methods Series 17. Los Angeles: Sage.

Fetterman, David M. (2013) *Ethnography: Step-by-Step* (3rd edition). Applied Social Research Methods Series 17. Los Angeles: Sage.

Gavioli, Laura (2012) Minimal responses in interpreter-mediated medical talk. In Claudio Baraldi and Laura Gavioli (eds) *Coordinating Participation in Dialogue Interpreting*, 201–228. Amsterdam: John Benjamins. https://doi.org/10.1075/btl.102.09gav

Hale, Sandra B. (2004) *The Discourse of Court Interpreting*. Amsterdam: John Benjamins. https://doi.org/10.1075/btl.52

Heritage, John and Paul Drew (1992) Analyzing talk at work: An introduction. In Paul Drew and John Heritage (eds) *Talk at Work: Interaction in Institutional Settings*, 3–65. Cambridge: Cambridge University Press.

Hill, Jane H. and Judith T. Irvine (eds) (1993) *Responsibility and Evidence in Oral Discourse*. Cambridge: Cambridge University Press.

Hsieh, Elaine and Soo Jung Hong (2010) Not all are desired: Providers' views on interpreters' emotional support for patients. *Patient Education and Counselling* 81 (2): 192–197. https://doi.org/10.1016/j.pec.2010.04.004

Metzger, Melanie (1999) *Sign Language Interpreting: Deconstructing the Myth of Neutrality*, 1–9. Washington, DC: Gallaudet University Press.

Meyer, Bernd (2012) *Ad hoc* interpreting for partially language-proficient patients: Participation in multilingual constellations. In Claudio Baraldi and Laura Gavioli (eds) *Coordinating Participation in Dialogue Interpreting*, 99–114. Amsterdam: John Benjamins. https://doi.org/10.1075/btl.102.05mey

Paradis, Michel (2000) Prerequisites for a study of neurolinguistic processes involved in simultaneous interpreting: A synopsis. In Birgitta E. Dimitrova and Kenneth Hyltenstam (eds) *Language Processing and Simultaneous Interpreting: Interdisciplinary Perspectives*, 17–24. Amsterdam: John Benjamins. https://doi.org/10.1075/btl.40.03par

Pollabauer, Sonja (2017) The interpreter's role. In UNHCR Austria (ed.) *Handbook for Interpreters in Asylum Procedures*, 50–69. Vienna: UNHCR Austria.

Roy, Cynthia B. (2000) *Interpreting as a Discourse Process*. New York: Oxford University Press.

Russo, Mariachiara (2011) Aptitude testing over the years. *Interpreting* 13 (1): 5–30. https://doi.org/10.1075/intp.13.1.02rus

Sarangi, Srikant (2012) Owning responsible actions/selves: Role-relational trajectories in counselling for childhood genetic testing. *Journal of Applied Linguistics and Professional Practice* 9 (3): 295–318. https://doi.org/10.1558/japl.v9i3.25743

Sawyer, David B. (2004) *Fundamental Aspects of Interpreter Education: Curriculum and Assessment*. Amsterdam: John Benjamins. https://doi.org/10.1075/btl.47

Solin, Anna and Jan-Ola Östman (2012) Introduction: Discourse and responsibility. *Journal of Applied Linguistics and Professional Practice* 9 (3): 287–294. https://doi.org/10.1558/japl.v9i3.20841

Teas Gill, Virginia and Douglas W. Maynard (2006) Explaining illness: Patients' proposals and physicians' responses. In John Heritage and Douglas W. Maynard (eds) *Communication in Medical Care: Interactions between Primary-Care Physicians and Patients*. Studies in International Sociolinguistics 20: 115–150. Cambridge: Cambridge University Press. https://doi.org/10.1017/CBO9780511607172.007

Valdés, Guadalupe, Christina Chávez, Claudia Angelelli, Dania García, Marisela González and Leisy Wyman (2003) The study of young interpreters: Methods, materials and analytical challenges. In Guadalupe Valdes (ed.) *Expanding Definitions of Giftedness: The Case of Young Interpreters from Immigrant Communities*, 99–118. Mahwah, NJ: Lawrence Erlbaum Associates. https://doi.org/10.4324/9781410607249-4

Wadensjö, Cecilia (1995) Dialogue interpreting and the distribution of responsibility. *Hermes Journal of Linguistics* 14: 111–129. https://doi.org/10.7146/hjlcb.v8i14.25098

Wadensjö, Cecilia (1998) *Interpreting as Interaction*. Harlow, UK: Addison Wesley Longman.

Claudia V. Angelelli is Professor and Chair in Multilingualism and Communication at Heriot-Watt University, Professor Emerita at San Diego State University and Visiting Professor at Beijing Foreign Studies University. Her work appears in journals such as *AAAL, EUJAL, Interpreting, IJSL, JALPP, Meta, MonTI, The Translator* and *TIS*. She is the author of *Revisiting* *the Interpreter's Role* (John Benjamins, 2004), *Medical Interpreting and Cross-cultural Communication* (Cambridge University Press, 2004) and *Medical Interpreting Explained* (Routledge, 2018). She is also guest editor of *The Sociological Turn in Translation and Interpreting Studies* (a special issue of *Translation and Interpreting Studies* [7:2], 2012) , *Translators and Interpreters: Geographic Displacement and Linguistic Consequences* (a special issue of the *International Journal of the Sociology of Language* [207], 2011) and *Minding the Gaps: Translation and Interpreting Studies in Academia* (a special issue of *Cuadernos de ALDEEU* [25], 2013) and the co-editor of *Testing and Assessment in Translation and Interpreting Studies* (John Benjamins, 2009) and *Researching Translation and Interpreting Studies* (Routledge, 2015). Address for correspondence: Department of Languages and Intercultural Studies, LINCS, School of Social Sciences, Heriot-Watt University, Henry Prais 2.03, Edinburgh Campus – EH14 4AS, UK. Email: c.angelelli@hw.ac.uk

3 Understanding interpreters' actions in context

Galina B. Bolden

3.1 Introduction

This article aims to examine how doctor–patient consultations shape (and are shaped by) interpreters' vocal and non-vocal conduct in ways that go beyond translation. I show that, like other participants, interpreters continuously monitor and analyze the unfolding interaction and make moment-by-moment decisions about their participation in it. The article draws on a larger conversation-analytic study of audio- and video-recorded consultations between English-speaking doctors, their Russian-speaking patients, and bilingual interpreters (*ad hoc* and professional) in a variety of medical settings (see Bolden 1998, 2000). Here, I present a microanalysis of two short segments to demonstrate that interpreters' participation in these interactions is not limited to translation. Instead, interpreters' actions – both what they say and their non-vocal conduct – are shaped by the demands of the interactional and medical activities the participants are engaged in.

Unlike a perceived view of interpreting as a process that involves a simple turn-by-turn translation of messages from one language to another (see the literature review below), this article aims to demonstrate that interpreting should be understood as an activity in its own right, coordinated with and embedded within ongoing activities. I show that what interpreters do or say in medical consultations is only partially, and sometimes hardly at all, limited to translating other people's talk. Interpreters' actions manifest a choice between several alternatives available to them at any particular time within the frame of the unfolding activity (see also Baraldi and Gavioli 2016). These alternatives, ranging from 'simply translating' between two languages to having an independent interactional position, embody interpreters' moment-by-moment decisions about what actions will be the most appropriate in a particular interactional environment. Interpreters' actions are thus organized in response to the demands of the unfolding medical activities.

Following a brief literature review and a description of the data and methodology, I examine (a) how an interpreter deals with a situation in which participants experience difficulties in understanding each other, and (b) how an interpreter participates in a physical examination activity that requires a close coordination of participants' bodily actions.

3.2 Literature review

The view of interpreting adopted in the present study contrasts with the traditional perception of interpreting as simply a means of conveying verbal messages between people who do not share a common language. It is often believed that interpreters are 'voice boxes' or 'translating machines' that (should) simply transmit messages between monolingual parties (for a discussion of this view, see, for example, Knapp-Potthoff and Knapp 1986; Roy 2000). Any deviations from this utterance-by-utterance translation may then be seen as interpreter errors (for a review of this perspective, see Pöchhacker 2004: 141–144).

This view of interpreting has, however, been challenged by empirical investigations into the work interpreters do. Studies of perceptions of interpreter roles held by interpreters, institutional agents, and clients and studies of actual interpreter-mediated interactions have both painted a much more complex picture of what interpreting consists of. For example, medical interpreters have been found to act as cultural brokers, patient advocates, institutional gate-keepers, helpers, co-therapists, and co-diagnosticians (e.g., Kaufert and Koolage 1984; Bolden 2000; Davidson 2000, 2001; Pöchhacker 2004; Leanza 2005; Valero-Garcés 2005; Merlini and Favaron 2005; Hsieh 2008; Rowland 2008; Raymond 2014a, 2014b) as well as to be involved in coordinating the flow of interaction (Wadensjö 1998; Bot 2005; Baraldi and Gavioli 2012). Overall, this research shows that an 'invisible' interpreter is more of a myth than a reality (Angelelli 2004).

The present study provides further support for this more complex view of what interpreting involves. Until recently, the majority of studies on medical interpreting have used survey instruments, interviews, or observations rather than audio-/video-recordings of interpreter-mediated consultations (for some recent developments in the field, see Baraldi and Gavioli 2012; Raymond 2014a, 2014b; Biagini *et al.* 2017). Moreover, even those studies that used video-recordings have paid little or no attention to interpreters' non-vocal conduct (but see, e.g., Wadensjö 2001; Pasquandrea 2011; Mason 2012; Davitti and Pasquandrea 2017). This paper advances the current understanding of interpreting practices by presenting a micro-analytic investigation of interpreters' verbal and nonverbal participation in actual medical consultations.

3.3 Data and method

The data for this study come from a corpus of video- and audio-recorded interpreter-mediated consultations between English-speaking doctors and Russian-speaking patients collected at a large hospital (11 audio-recorded encounters) and in a small optometrist's office (13 video-recorded consultations), both in the United Sates. The extracts analyzed here are drawn from two medical consultations: one was audio-recorded in the emergency room, the other video-recorded in an optometrist's office. In the hospital visit, a professionally trained hospital staff interpreter was employed; in the optometrist's office visit, an office assistant served as an *ad hoc* interpreter. Institutionally approved data collection and informed consent procedures were followed. The recorded data were transcribed and analyzed using the methodology of conversation analysis (Sidnell and Stivers 2013; Hepburn and Bolden 2017).

3.4 Analysis

The analysis section examines two common situations interpreters may find themselves in: managing difficulties in understanding, and coordinating a physical examination activity. Two case studies explicate the organization of interpreters' actions in these interactional contexts.

Managing trouble in interaction

A common expectation is that an interpreter's participation in interaction is limited to translating (in the next conversational turn) what one of the principal parties (i.e., the doctor or the patient) has just said. In order to live up to this norm, the interpreter needs to constantly monitor and analyze the principal parties' talk. Results of the interpreter's analysis may, however, reveal that what is said by one of the parties cannot simply be rendered into another language. For example, the talk to be translated may display its speaker's misunderstanding of the preceding interaction; or the speaker may use language the interpreter is unfamiliar with and, thus, may not be able to translate. In such situations the interpreter is forced to step outside of the 'translating machine' role and to engage in problem resolution (Wadensjö 1998; Raymond 2014b). In fact, failure to do so is likely to expand the misunderstanding and aggravate the situation.

While repairing problems of understanding, hearing, and speaking is common in any type of talk-in-interaction (e.g., Schegloff *et al.* 1977), the type of trouble that will be analyzed here is specific to interpreter-mediated communication, since it has to do with a problem in translation. Specifically, the problem arises when the interpreter is unable to provide an adequate translation of an utterance produced by the patient. The analysis will show that the interpreter takes an active role in dealing with and resolving this interactional problem. As a result, the interpreter's orientation to her normative responsibilities as a translator compels her to act in ways that are divergent from doing translation *per se*. Thus, the interpreter's participation in this segment is not constrained by the 'voice box' view of interpreting but by the requirements of the unfolding interactional environment – specifically, the unfolding repair sequence.

Case Study 1: 'They wouldn't know Latin?'

The segment of interaction analyzed here comes from a medical consultation in an emergency room (ER). An elderly Russian woman was brought to the ER with an acute heart problem. At the start of Excerpt 1a, two physicians are attending to her, and a professional staff interpreter has been called in. What makes this case particularly challenging is that the patient herself is a retired cardiologist. Her expertise in the field is made relevant in the segment of interaction analyzed here. The excerpt is taken from the history-taking part of the consultation, during which the physicians discuss with the patient her prior medical problems, including a heart attack she had several years earlier. Just prior to this segment, one of the physicians (D1) inquires if the patient (P) remembers whether she had an electrocardiogram (EKG) done at the time of the first heart attack.

The first question in this segment (lines 1 and 3) refers to the results of that EKG. (The transcription conventions are explained in the Appendix.)

Excerpt 1a: ER. D1 = Doctor; D2 = Doctor 2; I = Interpreter; P = Patient

1 D1: Do you remember if you had any
2 P: (O[:)/
PRT
(Oh)
3 D1: [queue: waves in (.) blee
4 [twee¿
5 I: [U vas byli kuab[ra:znye
with you were que-like
Did you have Q like
6 P: [Blakada levaj
blockade left
Blockade of the left
7 levaj vn: n:ozhki puchka
left leg bundle
left bl: leg of
8 [agibal'nava=
rounding
the rounding bundle
9 I: [hhh.
10 P: =levaj vetvi puchka Gi,sa/
left branch bundle His'
of the left branch of His' bundle
11 (0.5)
12 I: Heh-heh-heh-heh-
13 [hehhh [£that's goo:d.£
14 P: [Oj/ [tr(h)udna perevesti/
PRT hard translate
Oy it's hard to translate
15 I: O:h. .hhh

Repair initiation: The doctor's question (lines 1 and 3) is designed to elicit a specific piece of technical information about the patient's EKG. The patient's response (lines 6–10) is formulated in very technical terms that the interpreter, who is not a medical expert, finds problematic for translation. The interpreter's difficulty with the patient's utterance is made public through her laughter (line 12) and a metalinguistic comment in English: *£that's goo:d.£* (line 13). The patient understands the laughter as signaling a problem in translating her response, as evident in her subsequent comment: *Oy it's hard to translate* (line 14). Thus, in lines 12–13 the interpreter foregrounds the difficulty with translating the patient's response and, by doing so, initiates repair on the patient's talk. The interpreter's participation in the interaction is from now on structured by the sequential constraints of the unfolding repair sequence.

Repair resolution: Repair sequences are, by definition, sequences during which the activity in the midst of which they occur is put on hold until the trouble is resolved (Schegloff *et al.* 1977). Given the preference for progressivity in conversation (Stivers and Robinson 2006; Heritage 2007) – that is, parties' orientation to advancing conversational activities – participants strive to resolve interactional problems quickly, i.e., with least disruption to the main course of action. This may be particularly true of interpreter-mediated interaction, since using an interpreter necessarily entails delays for parties who do not share a common language. A repair sequence in an interpreter-mediated interaction may thus seriously impede the progress of the main activity. An examination of the repair sequence in Excerpt 1b demonstrates that the interpreter continuously analyzes the ongoing talk for how to resolve the problem in interaction so as to minimize the disruption to the main course of action. As the interaction continues, the interpreter attempts to translate the patient's problematic utterance (line 17).

Excerpt 1b: ER

16 P: ([ )
17 I: [khe-khe Like a le:ft bra:nch or
18 P: Ani latyn' ne zna¿jut da/=
they Latin not know yes
They wouldn't know Latin right
19 I: =You know [Latin?
20 D2: [That's (.) bundle branch?=
21 I: =Znajut/[Znajut/<Esli vy skazhite]=
know know if you say
They do they do. If you say it
22 P: [Znajut latyn da?/]
know latin yes
They know Latin right
23 I: =po laty,ne/ da/
in Latin yes
in Latin yes
24 P: Da/ .h gipertrafija
Yes hypertonia
Yes hypertonia

25 levova zheludochka (sjuda)
left ventricle here
of the left ventricle
26 I: .h(hypertonia)of the le:ft va:lve,
27 (1.2)

The interpreter's attempt at the translation (line 17) is abandoned as soon as the patient asks whether the doctors would know Latin (line 18). Given the sequential position of this question within the repair sequence, the question is clearly not just a request for information but also a proposal of a possible repair resolution. The interpreter, after translating the question into English (line 19), provides a response that attends to both the informational aspect of the question (*they do they do* in line 21) and to its interactional import (*if you say it in Latin yes* in lines 21 and 23). Without a visual record of the interaction, it is impossible to say whether the first part of the interpreter's answer (*they do, they do*) is the interpreter's own position or a verbalization of the doctors' non-vocal cues. However, in the absence of a verbal response from the doctors, it is clear that at least the second part of the utterance demonstrates the interpreter's own analysis of the interactional import of the patient's question.

The interpreter's ongoing analysis of the unfolding activity and her orientation to furthering its progress are also evident in how she handles a situation in which two alternative courses of action are proposed. Line 18 is a repair resolution proposal put forward by the patient: *They wouldn't know Latin?*. If accepted, the repair will be done through the patient's restatement (in Latin) of her initial response to the doctor's question (from lines 5–10). This is in fact what eventually happens: *hypertonia of the left ventricle* (lines 24–25).

In line 20, however, one of the doctors takes a different tack in solving the problem by proffering a candidate understanding of the interpreter's turn in line 17: *That's (.) bundle branch?*. This is clearly an inferior method for dealing with the problem in this interactional environment, since it may lead to an extended sequence of attempts by the doctor to guess the patient's meaning – attempts to which the interpreter may not be able to respond to adequately, due to lack of technical expertise. By choosing neither to respond nor translate the doctor's turn (but rather respond to the patient in lines 22 and 24), the interpreter prevents this course of repair resolution from developing. The interpreter's actions thus demonstrate her independent analysis of the ongoing activity. Specifically, the interpreter evaluates different means of repair resolution and chooses the course of action that will resolve repair most efficiently.

Further evidence for this comes from subsequent talk in Excerpt 1c.

Excerpt 1c: ER

28 P: [( )
29 D2: [Of the left wa:ll?
30 I: Yeah
31 P: I budi-=
PRT will
And will-
32 D2: =( ) left lea: [f?
33 P: [I: saver[shenna=
PRT completely
And completely
34 I: [Yeah
35 P: =atsuctvaval er zubec/ Er/
was-absent R peak R
absent was the R-wave. The R
36 I: R:- (.) R-wave was [a:bsent=
37 D1: [hm-hm,
38 I: =if tha[t >makes [any sense to you<
39 P: [Ot V-
from V
From V-
40 D2: [Yeah.(.) Yeah, yeah.
41 D1: [Yeah
42 P: [at ve adin,/ da ve chetyr[e/
from V one to V four
from V one to V four.
43 D1: [Hm-mmh:,

Just prior to this part of the segment, the interpreter provides a translation of the patient's response: *.h(Hypertonia) of the le:ft va:lve,* (line 26). One of the doctors (D2) apparently finds the interpreter's translation problematic and proffers candidate understandings of that translation (lines 29 and 32). The interpreter's participation in the interaction as an independent social actor is underscored by the fact that she responds to these candidate understandings instead of translating them into Russian (lines 30 and 34). In this way, the interpreter demonstrates her analysis of the doctor's turn as being directed to the problems in *her translation* and *not* in the patient's original utterance.

Moreover, when the patient offers another piece of information that can potentially clarify her prior utterance (lines 33 and 35), the interpreter translates it into English (line 36). The translation is followed by a gloss (*if that >makes any sense to you<* – line 38), which invites the two doctors to assess the translation on the basis of its comprehensibility. At the same time, the utterance shows that the interpreter chose this way of repair resolution in spite of the fact that she did not understand the utterance's meaning.[1] The interpreter's decision to switch tracks in the repair sequence demonstrates her understanding that the previous route via candidate understandings (offered by one of the doctors) has not been productive. The interpreter's decision turns out to be the right one, as we can see from the two doctors' affirmative reaction (lines 40 and 41).

Thus, the analysis of this segment of interaction has demonstrated that the interpreter's participation in the ongoing activity is not limited to translating the talk of the other parties. In fact, the interpreter's orientation to her responsibilities as an interpreter compels her to step outside the strictly translating role (cf. Raymond 2014b). In addition, the interpreter's departures from doing translation demonstrate the interpreter's systematic orientation to the demands of the particular unfolding interactional environment – in this case, the repair sequence.

Coordinating a physical examination

Interpreters may step out of their role as translators of verbal messages not only when dealing with understanding or translation problems, but for a variety of other reasons. Here I examine another recurrent situation that necessitates more than translating: a routine physical examination activity. A close analysis of a segment of interaction will demonstrate that the interpreter does not simply reproduce other people's talk, but acts – both vocally and visibly – in ways that display her 'reflexive awareness' of the changing contextual contingencies (Goodwin 2000). The interpreter, as a competent social actor, continuously analyzes the unfolding interaction and adapts her behavior (including speech, gaze, body movement, gestures, and other bodily actions) to the immediately relevant features of context. I show that the interpreter's involvement in the physical examination is better understood by reference to the ongoing medical activity, rather than by reference to the other parties' talk.

Case Study 2: 'We're checking pressure in the eye'

This interaction comes from a corpus of data collected at an optometrist's office. Four participants are present: the patient (P) and her husband (H), the doctor (D), and the interpreter (I). The patient, her husband, and the interpreter are Armenian immigrants to the US and speak Russian and Armenian. The interpreter, who is fluent in English and who acts as interpreter for Russian and Armenian patients, also works as an office manager at this doctor's office. The target segment comes from a routine eye examination. In this segment, the doctor conducts a glaucoma test, which measures eye pressure with an instrument called the tonometer (see Figure 3.1). During the test, the patient needs to position her head on the frame of the tonometer with the chin on the chin rest and the forehead against the forehead rest. The doctor examines the eye through the eyepiece.

Activity boundaries: The glaucoma test has distinct interactional boundaries within a medical consultation. It starts with the doctor positioning the tonometer in front of the patient and it stops when the goal of the activity (measuring eye pressure in both eyes) is fulfilled and the

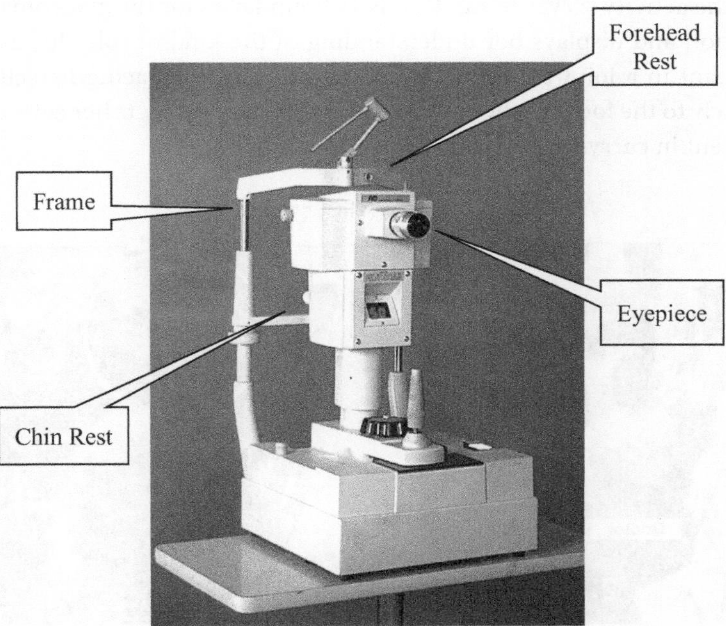

Figure 3.1 The tonometer.

tonometer is returned to its initial position. In the segment analyzed here the interpreter plays a key role in managing the boundaries of this activity.

Interlocutors' participation in face-to-face interaction is clearly shaped by the kind of access (visual and otherwise) they have to the current focal activity (Goodwin 1996, 2000). Parties who are proximate to the focus of the activity usually have more ways of engaging in it (through both talk and physical action). Thus, participants' positioning *vis-à-vis* the physical focus of the activity may serve to project their involvement in it. At the same time, participants' movement within the setting may display their understanding of what the focus of the activity is and what kind of involvement on their part is expected.

In this data segment, the interpreter's positioning during the glaucoma test is markedly different from her positioning during the rest of the medical consultation. While throughout the consultation, the interpreter sits at the back of the room behind the doctor, during the glaucoma test she gets up and positions herself next to the patient in a way that provides her both visual and physical access to the patient and to the tonometer (see Figure 3.2). After the examination is over, the interpreter again moves to the back of the room. Thus, the interpreter's positioning *vis-à-vis* the focus of the activity serves to mark activity boundaries for the glaucoma examination and displays her understanding of the kind of role she, as a participant in a joint action, will play. Specifically, by placing herself proximately to the focus of the activity, the interpreter projects her active involvement in carrying it out.[2]

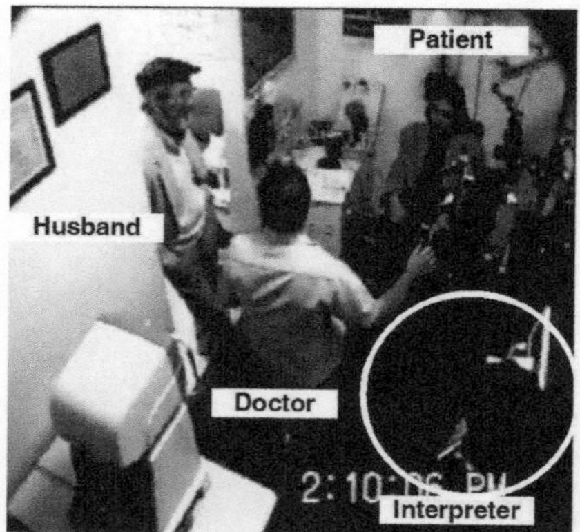

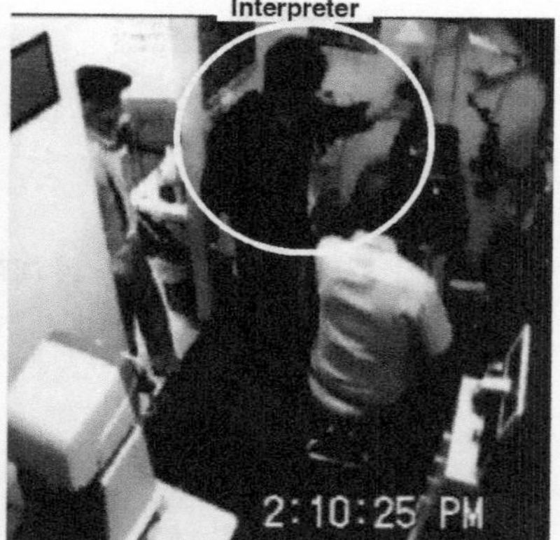

Figure 3.2 The interpreter's location before and during the test.

Launching a request sequence: A closer examination of the interpreter's actions at the activity boundary shows that her actions demonstrate her independent analysis of the unfolding medical activity and are timed *vis-à-vis* that activity. As mentioned earlier, before the examination can begin, the doctor needs to rearrange various instruments in a way that would enable him to conduct the test. Specifically, the doctor needs to move the tonometer right in front of the patient, adjust the height of the patient's chair so that the patient is aligned with the tonometer, and move behind the tonometer so that he can see through the eyepiece.

In Excerpt 2a, while the doctor carries out these tasks (lines 1–14 below) the interpreter sits in the back of the room and is visibly disengaged from the activity up to line 20, when she begins to get up from her chair.

Excerpt 2a: Eye Examination. D = Doctor; H = Husband; I = Interpreter; P = Patient

1 D: Oka:y no:w:,
2 (0.6)
3 H: (Gavarjat) Doctar/
they+say doctor
(They say) Doctor
4 (1.0)
5 D: Pardon me?
6 H: Ah-heh-heh-heh-heh-heh
7 .hhh heh-heh-[heh-heh
8 D: [I need he:r to:
9 (0.6)
10 H: .hh
11 (2.5)
12 H: *( )*
13 I: Huh-huh,
14 H: Heh-heh
15 (0.4)
16 H: [heh-heh
17 D: [I need'er tuh put her chi:n,
18 (0.2)
19 I: Oke::j eh: pastafte vash podb-
okay put your ch-
Okay uh put your ch-
⇑#1
20 [podbarodak sjuda,/
chin here
chin here
[((I begins to stand up))
⇑#2
21 (0.4)

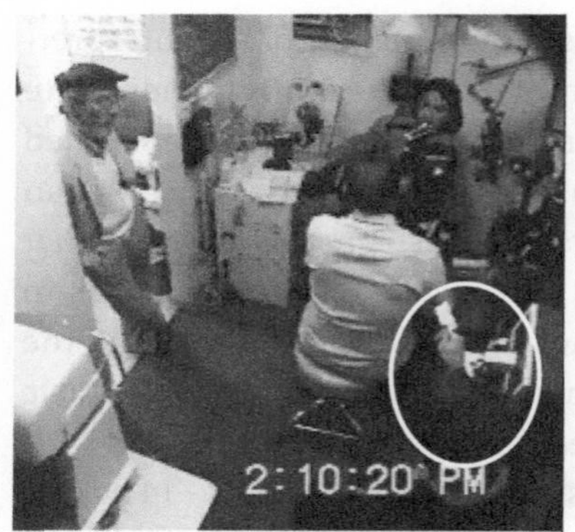

#1

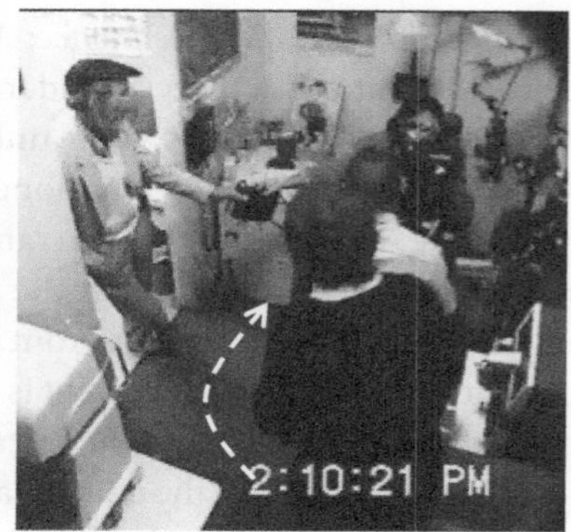

#2

During lines 19–21, the interpreter gets up and moves towards the patient's chair, where she has better access to the focus of the activity. What prompts the interpreter to change her location (and, therefore, her participation status) at that particular time? In general, requests make compliance (or refusal) conditionally relevant, with compliance being the preferred response since it promotes the accomplishment of the activity in progress (Schegloff 2007). The work of furthering the activity is not only the business of the recipient of a request, but also of its issuer, who should aim to issue the request when compliance is possible. During a glaucoma test, the patient cannot position her chin on the tonometer frame until the instrument is right in front of her. This is a contingency both the doctor and the interpreter are oriented to. While the doctor initiates the request (addressed to the interpreter) to position the patient's head on the tonometer frame (*I need he:r to:* – line 8), he is oriented to the fact that the patient is unable to comply with the instruction until he arranges the instruments involved in the activity. So even though the doctor launches the instruction for the patient to move into the exam position in line 8, he suspends the turn in progress until he is able to attend to all relevant medical instruments (up until line 17).

The interpreter is also oriented to this contingency and does not start translating the doctor's request until the doctor is just about ready for the patient to comply with it – even though she has multiple opportunities to do so. Note especially that, at line 8, the doctor begins to solicit the interpreter's assistance in this task (by using the third person reference form 'her' to refer to the patient); yet, the interpreter does not move or start translating the doctor's instruction, which is indicative of her own

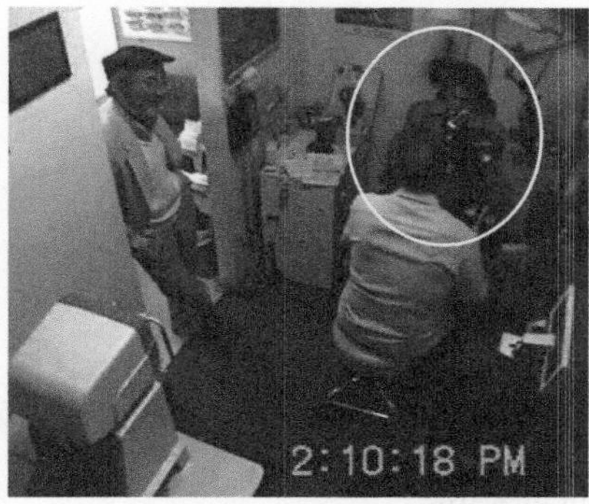

Figure 3.3 Eye examination, end of line 17.

analysis of the activity in progress. The instruments are close to being properly positioned at the completion of line 17, as shown in Figure 3.3 (note that the tonometer is almost in front of the patient's face).

It is at this point that the interpreter produces a request for the patient to move into the examination position (lines 19–20). Notably, this is not simply a translation of the doctor's words but an action that displays the interpreter's analysis of the ongoing activity. In fact, the interpreter expands the doctor's verbal request in several important ways. First, during the production of the turn, the interpreter points towards the tonometer (at arrow #1) and then gets up and starts moving in the direction of the patient (at arrow #2). Second, in her translation the interpreter provides an indexical location reference *here* which was absent in the doctor's turn in line 2. The referent of *here* (i.e. the chin rest) is disambiguated when the interpreter is in the position next to the tonometer where she can point to the appropriate location (Goodwin 2003).

Positioning the patient's head: The interpreter's participation in the activity as an autonomous social actor is underscored in Excerpt 2b, during which the interpreter and the doctor cooperate in positioning the patient's head on the tonometer frame. The interpreter starts directing the patient as soon as she reaches the tonometer, and by the end of the segment, the patient's head is properly placed on the frame.

Excerpt 2b: Eye examination

22 I: [i my]
and we
And we're

23 D: [Have'er] chin re [sted]

24 I: [pra]verjaem
check
checking

25 [davlen]ie v glazu/]
pressure in eye
pressure in the eye

26 D: [forehead]up again]st the to:p.
⇑#3

27 (0.5)

28 I: eta samae uh:: vperët/
and this very uh forward
A:nd so uh:: Forward
⇑#4 ⇑#5

29 Golavu vperë,t/vperët/ V-net=
head forward forward no
Head forward forward No
⇑#6

30 D: [=Okay

31 I: [vot eta chast' sjuda/
PRT this part here
This part ((goes)) here

32 (0.4)

33 D: °Good°=

34 I: =Tak/
PRT
=Like this
⇑#7

35 (0.8)
⇑#8

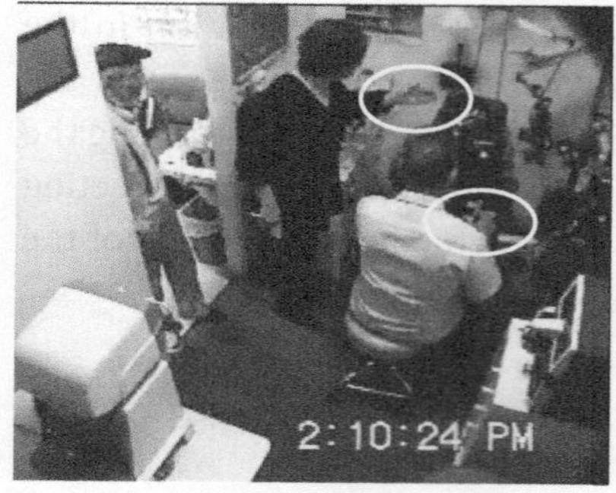

#3

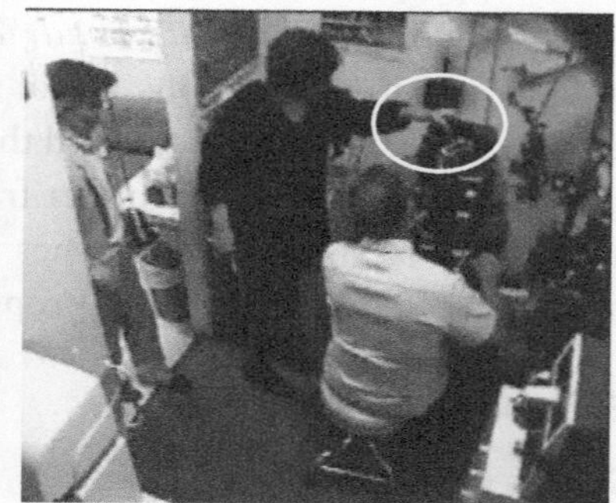

#4

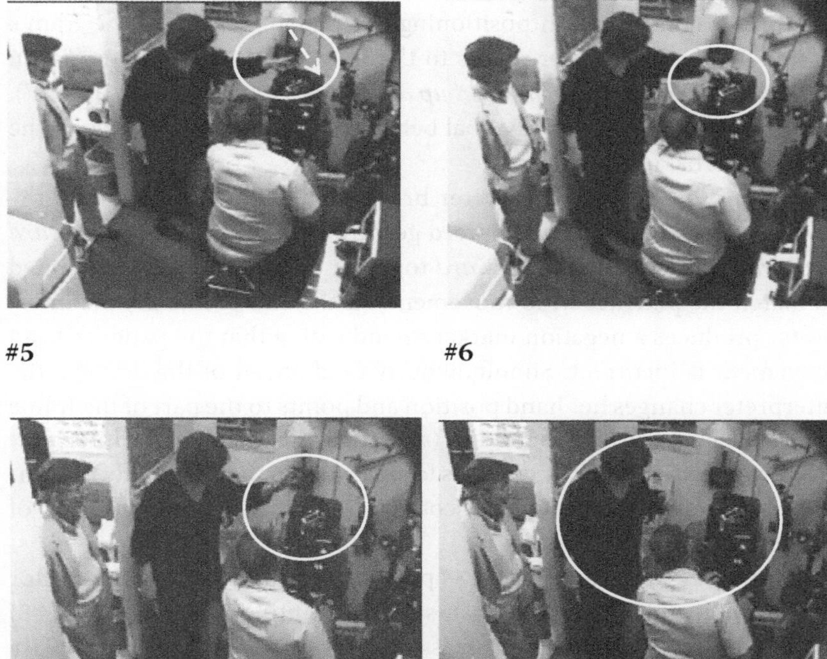

#5 #6

#7 #8

During the first several seconds of this segment (lines 22–26), the interpreter and the doctor are engaged in carrying out two different tasks simultaneously. While the interpreter directs the patient's head, the doctor manipulates the controls on the tonometer (#3). It should be noted that the interpreter's turn, *And we're checking pressure in the eye* (lines 22 and 24–25), is not a translation of anything the doctor has said, but the interpreter's own formulation of the goal of the examination. This utterance shows that the interpreter monitors, analyzes, and partitions the ongoing medical examination into recognizable parts (such as the glaucoma test). The interpreter's use of the pronoun *we* also suggests that the interpreter sees herself as the doctor's collaborator. Furthermore, the doctor's instructions (lines 17 and 23) are designed in such a way as to portray the interpreter as an assistant. In fact, throughout the glaucoma test, the interpreter acts as a medical paraprofessional rather than a language translator. In the next several seconds, the doctor and the interpreter collaborate in positioning the patient's head on the frame. In line 28, the interpreter points to the frame of the tonometer (#4) in response to the doctor's *forehead up against the t:op.* direction (line 27). Thus, the interpreter's non-verbal behavior is directly responsive to the doctor's verbal instructions.

In lines 28–29, the interpreter brings her hand to the back of the patient's head and makes a forward gesture (#5): *Forward head forward forward.* The repetition of *forward* together with this gesture are timed to match the patient's head movement. At the end of line 29, the interpreter produces a negation marker *no* indicating that the patient's head movement is incorrect. Simultaneously (and ahead of the doctor), the interpreter changes her hand position and points to the part of the frame where the patient's head should go (#6). Thus, the design of the interpreter's turn together with her gestures form an action that is directly responsive to the immediate features of context (in this case, the positioning of the patient's head).

As soon as the patient's head is positioned properly, both the doctor and the interpreter simultaneously stop the pointing gestures (#7 and #8) and produce sequence-closing assessment tokens: *Good* (line 33) and *Like this* (line 34) (Schegloff 2007). The interpreter's physical disengagement from the current action (withdrawing her hand) and her verbal response (the sequence closing token) demonstrate that the interpreter analyzes the progress of the activity (whether or not the patient's head is positioned properly) and designs her actions to match it.

To summarize, the analysis of this part of the interaction has shown that the interpreter plays an active role in conducting the physical examination. The interpreter's actions, both those that are directly responsive to the doctor's verbal instructions and those that are independent of them, demonstrate the interpreter's own analysis of the progress of the physical examination activity.

Reassuring the patient: Aside from positioning the patient's body properly *vis-à-vis* relevant artifacts, physical examinations of various sorts often involve tasks that are designed to ensure patients' cooperation in the examination. For example, patients may be warned about the discomforts they will experience during the test. Such warnings are often necessary to successfully accomplish the examination, since they not only reassure the patient but also secure his/her proper participation in the activity (e.g., Heath 1986). My analysis of several glaucoma examinations conducted by the same doctor with English-speaking patients has shown that reassuring the patient is one of the tasks the doctor routinely carries out. For example, during one recorded examination the doctor says: *When I press the button you'll feel a puff of air but nothing will touch the eye, it's just air.* In the interpreter-mediated interaction shown in Excerpt 2c, the interpreter is the one who provides the reassurance:

Excerpt 2c: Eye Examination

36 I: Eta tol'ka vozdux/
this only air uh
This is just air
37 Eh: ne bojtes'/
not be-afraid
Don't be afraid
38 D: Just look str[aight ahead.
39 I: [Et` ne bol'na/
this not hurt
This won't hurt
40 D: [(°Don't move °)
41 I: [<Posmatrite v tochku/
look at dot
Look at the dot
42 Tam kr:asnaja tochku uvidete¿/
there red dot will+see
You'll see there a red dot
((the exam continues))

The utterance in lines 36–37 and 39, which serves to reassure the patient, is produced on the interpreter's initiative, unprompted by any talk on the part of the doctor. The interpreter then continues to direct the patient to look *at the dot* (line 41), which is responsive to but different from the doctor's instruction to look *straight ahead* (line 38). Furthermore, the interpreter, with no prompting from the doctor, provides an explanation for this directive (line 42). Overall, the interpreter's involvement in this part of the examination further instantiates a division of labor between the doctor and the interpreter that results from the interpreter's independent analysis of the ongoing activity and her competent participation in it.

To summarize, the analysis of this interaction has demonstrated that the interpreter's verbal and bodily actions during the eye examination cannot be understood by reference to the talk produced by other parties, but rather primarily by reference to the ongoing activity. For example, the interpreter's online behavior displays her orientation to activity boundaries and reflects her moment-by-moment evaluation of the relevant contextual features (such as the other parties' engagement with the pertinent artifacts). In other words, the interpreter continuously monitors and analyzes all relevant components of the unfolding interaction, and not just the other parties' talk.

The glaucoma test examined here is a complex activity that requires precise coordination of people (the doctor, the patient, and the interpreter) and artifacts (parts of the measuring instrument, the chairs, etc.). Since patients typically have little experience with this medical procedure, the interpreter's involvement as a competent social actor may be required in order for the physical examination to run smoothly and effectively. Furthermore, the glaucoma test is an extremely standardized activity, during which the participants follow an orderly plan of action that is familiar not only to the doctor but also to the interpreter, who (in this case) has participated in many such consultations. Due to the precision this examination requires and its routine and relatively fixed character, participants are limited in what they can appropriately do within the frame of the activity. Hence while the interpreter's participation in this physical examination activity appears unconstrained by other people's talk, it is in fact constrained by the exigencies of the activity itself.

3.5 Discussion and conclusion

The presented analysis has demonstrated that interpreting is a complex activity that cannot be understood as simply the rendering of other people's talk into another language. In fact, through a micro-analytic investigation of interpreter-mediated interactions, we have seen that what interpreters do or say is *not*, in the first instance, shaped by other people's talk but by interpreters' own independent analysis of the ongoing activity and the constraints it poses on the participants (cf. Levinson 1992). This study thus provides further evidence for the view that interpreters conduct themselves not as translating machines but as full-fledged social actors who make moment-by-moment decisions about their verbal and bodily actions (e.g., Angelelli 2004; Baraldi and Gavioli 2016).

While the findings presented here are based on an analysis of only two short segments of interaction, it is clear that at least some of the conclusions could be generalized. In particular, from this and other studies of interpreter conduct, it is evident that researchers cannot limit themselves to comparing interpreters' utterances to utterances they are, presumably, translations of and then classifying them on the basis of how closely these utterances correspond to their originals. Such an approach blends a wide range of divergent interactional phenomena without providing a reasonable explanation for the interpreter's actions. Neither can the analysis be limited to studying interpreters' talk in isolation from the activity it is a part of. We have seen, for example, that the interpreter's bodily actions may be as important as talk in coordinating interaction between a patient and a medical professional. Further research on interpreting in a variety of settings and for a variety of activities is needed to elucidate details on how different activity systems (such as medial history taking, physical examination, treatment recommendation) shape the interpreter's participation in the interaction. However, it is already apparent that for an adequate account of interpreting as a form of participation, it needs to be analyzed as a situated, locally organized activity embedded in a particular setting. Overall, this study furthers our understanding of interpreting as a situated activity and highlights the necessity of paying close analytic attention to the organization and unfolding of the courses of action interpreters serve to advance, within particular situational constraints.

This study may also have practical implications, especially for interpreter training. Interpreter-training programs generally prescribe that interpreters limit their involvement to translating words of the others parties. Yet, an analysis of actual interpreter-mediated interactions, such as those examined here, shows that this view may be impractical and, at times, even detrimental. The first case study, in which the interpreter actively manages interactional problems, indicates, for example, that interpreters might be better served if they are trained in how to deal with and repair interactional problems (for example, via guided data sessions, as discussed in Davitti and Pasquandrea 2014a). The second case study, in which the interpreter acts as a medical paraprofessional during an optometric examination, suggests that interpreters should, at least, be alerted to the fact that their non-vocal conduct is an important communicative resource that impacts the organization of interaction (see also Wadensjö 2001; Davitti and Pasquandrea 2014a). The empirical results reported here and elsewhere (Bolden 2000) indicate that interpreters may benefit from training in what constitutes appropriate participation in the interaction and what does not. While interpreters' active involvement in the interaction may be beneficial or even necessary in some circumstances (as discussed here), in other contexts, such involvement may negatively impact communication between medical professionals and their patients (see, e.g., Bolden 2000). Overall, this research points to tremendous benefits of incorporating authentic materials into interpreter education (Davitti and Pasquandrea 2014b).

Appendix: Transcription conventions

The transcripts employ conversation analytic transcription conventions (Hepburn and Bolden 2017). To represent Russian, the first line of the transcript shows transliterated Russian speech (see Bolden 2008 for an explication of the transliteration system); the second line is a word-for-word translation into English; the third line is idiomatic translation into English. The standard transcription conventions used are provided here.

.	falling intonation
,	continuing intonation
?	rising intonation
[	the point at which speakers start to talk in overlap
=	no time lapses between the latched utterances
(number)	silence measured in seconds
(.)	a micropause – silence under 0.2 second
:	stretching of the preceding sound
-	a cut-off sound
underline	stress or emphasis on the underlined sound or word
CAPITAL	especially loud talk
>word<	compressed or rushed speech
£word£	smiley voice
hhh	exhalation
.hh	inhalation
(h)	laugh tokens or breathing sounds during talk
((comment))	transcriber's comments
(text)	possible, uncertain hearing
( )	something is said but no hearing can be achieved
PRT	"particle"

For Russian, the following modifications to the above standard conventions are made:

, ? placed after the syllable carrying the distinct intonation contour (comma or questioning intonation) that will be actualized at the unit boundary

/ unit boundary. If no intonation symbol is placed in the preceding unit, it marks default, somewhat falling pitch contour

./ marks final pitch drop that is larger that the default, unmarked pitch drop

Notes

1 The gloss also lends evidence to the observation that the problem the interpreter experiences is not necessarily (or primarily) a problem of understanding but a problem of translation. Even though it is, of course, desirable for interpreters to understand the meaning of what they translate, this example demonstrates that it is not always required.

2 In contrast, the husband remains at the periphery throughout the consultation (at the doorway – see Figure 3.2), which is indicative of his non-involvement in the focal activity. Note as well that the husband steps a bit farther back out of the room during the glaucoma test, thus yielding to the interpreter (compare the two pictures in Figure 3.2).

References

Angelelli, Claudia V. (2004) *Medical Interpreting and Cross-Cultural Communication*. Cambridge: Cambridge University Press. https://doi.org/10.1017/CBO9780511486616

Baraldi, Claudio and Laura Gavioli (eds) (2012) *Coordinating Participation in Dialogue Interpreting*. Philadelphia: John Benjamins. https://doi.org/10.1075/btl.102

Baraldi, Claudio and Laura Gavioli (2016) On professional and non-professional interpreting in healthcare services: The case of intercultural mediators. *European Journal of Applied Linguistics* 4 (1): 33–55. https://doi.org/10.1515/eujal-2015-0026

Biagini, Marta, Elena Davitti and Annalisa Sandrelli (2017) Participation in interpreter-mediated interaction: Shifting along a multidimensional continuum. *Journal of Pragmatics* 107: 87–90. https://doi.org/10.1016/j.pragma.2016.11.001

Bolden, Galina B. (1998) *Practices of Medical Interpreting: An Interactional Account.* Unpublished Master's dissertation, University of California, Los Angeles.

Bolden, Galina B. (2000) Towards understanding practices of medical interpreting: Interpreters' involvement in history taking. *Discourse Studies* 2 (4): 387–419. https://doi.org/10.1177/1461445600002004001

Bolden, Galina B. (2008) Reopening Russian conversations: The discourse particle *-to* and the negotiation of interpersonal accountability in closings. *Human Communication Research* 34 (1): 99–136. https://doi.org/10.1111/j.1468-2958.2007.00315.x

Bot, Hanneke (2005) Dialogue interpreting as a special case of reported speech. *Interpreting* 7 (2): 237–261. https://doi.org/10.1075/intp.7.2.06bot

Davidson, Brad (2000) The interpreter as institutional gatekeeper: The social-linguistic role of interpreters in Spanish-English medical discourse. *Journal of Sociolinguistics* 4 (3): 379–405. https://doi.org/10.1111/1467-9481.00121

Davidson, Brad (2001) Questions in cross-linguistic medical encounters: The role of the hospital interpreter. *Anthropological Quarterly* 74 (4): 170–178. https://doi.org/10.1353/anq.2001.0035

Davitti, Elena and Sergio Pasquandrea (2014a) Enhancing research-led interpreter education: An exploratory study in applied conversation analysis. *The Interpreter and Translator Trainer* 8 (3): 374–398. https://doi.org/10.1080/1750399X.2014.972650

Davitti, Elena and Sergio Pasquandrea (2014b) Guest editorial. *The Interpreter and Translator Trainer* 8 (3): 329–335. https://doi.org/10.1080/1750399X.2014.973143

Davitti, Elena and Sergio Pasquandrea (2017) Embodied participation: What multimodal analysis can tell us about interpreter-mediated encounters in pedagogical settings. *Journal of Pragmatics* 107: 105–128. https://doi.org/10.1016/j.pragma.2016.04.008

Goodwin, Charles (1996) Transparent vision. In Elinor Ochs, Emanuel A. Schegloff and Sandra A. Thompson (eds) *Interaction and Grammar*, 370–404. Cambridge: Cambridge University Press. https://doi.org/10.1017/CBO9780511620874.008

Goodwin, Charles (2000) Action and embodiment within situated human interaction. *Journal of Pragmatics* 32 (10): 1489–1522. https://doi.org/10.1016/S0378-2166(99)00096-X

Goodwin, Charles (2003) Pointing as situated practice. In Sotaro Kita (ed.) *Pointing: Where Language, Culture and Cognition Meet*, 217–241. Mahwah, NJ: Lawrence Erlbaum Associates.

Heath, Christian (1986) *Body Movement and Speech in Medical Interaction.* Cambridge: Cambridge University Press. https://doi.org/10.1017/CBO9780511628221

Hepburn, Alexa and Galina B. Bolden (2017) *Transcribing for Social Research.* London: Sage. https://doi.org/10.4135/9781473920460

Heritage, John (2007) Intersubjectivity and progressivity in references to persons (and places). In Tanya Stivers and N. J. Enfield (eds) *Person Reference in Interaction: Linguistic, Cultural and Social Perspectives,* 255–280. Cambridge: Cambridge University Press.

Hsieh, Elaine (2008) 'I am not a robot!': Interpreters' views of their roles in health care settings. *Qualitative Health Research* 18 (10): 1367–1383. https://doi.org/10.1177/1049732308323840

Kaufert, Joseph M. and William W. Koolage (1984) Role conflict among 'culture brokers': The experience of native Canadian medical interpreters. *Social Science & Medicine* 18 (3): 283–286. https://doi.org/10.1016/0277-9536(84)90092-3

Knapp-Potthoff, Annelie and Karlfried Knapp (1986) Interweaving two discourses: The difficult task of the non-professional interpreter. In Juliane House and Shoshana Blum-Kulka (eds) *Interlingual and Intercultural Communication: Discourse and Cognition in Translation and Second Language Acquisition Studies,* 151–168. New York: Mouton.

Leanza, Yvan (2005) Roles of community interpreters in pediatrics as seen by interpreters, physicians and researchers. *Interpreting* 7 (2): 167–192. https://doi.org/10.1075/intp.7.2.03lea

Levinson, Stephen C. (1992) Activity types and language. In Paul Drew and John Heritage (eds) *Talk at Work: Interaction in Institutional Settings,* 66–100. Cambridge: Cambridge University Press.

Mason, Ian (2012) Gaze, positioning and identity in interpreter-mediated dialogues. In Claudio Baraldi and Laura Gavioli (eds) *Coordinating Participation in Dialogue Interpreting,* 177–199. Amsterdam: John Benjamins. https://doi.org/10.1075/btl.102.08mas

Merlini, Raffaela and Roberta Favaron (2005) Examining the 'voice of interpreting' in speech pathology. *Interpreting* 7 (2): 263–302. https://doi.org/10.1075/intp.7.2.07mer

Pasquandrea, Sergio (2011) Managing multiple actions through multimodality: Doctors' involvement in interpreter-mediated interactions. *Language in Society* 40 (4): 455–481. https://doi.org/10.1017/S0047404511000479

Pöchhacker, Franz (2004) *Introducing Interpreting Studies.* London: Routledge. https://doi.org/10.4324/9780203504802

Raymond, Chase W. (2014a) Conveying information in the interpreter-mediated medical visit: The case of epistemic brokering. *Patient Education and Counseling* 97 (1): 38–46. https://doi.org/10.1016/j.pec.2014.05.020

Raymond, Chase W. (2014b) Epistemic brokering in the interpreter-mediated medical visit: Negotiating 'patient's side' and 'doctor's side' knowledge. *Research on Language and Social Interaction* 47 (4): 426–446. https://doi.org/10.1080/08351813.2015.958281

Rowland, Michael L. (2008) Enhancing communication in dental clinics with linguistically different patients. *Journal of Dental Education* 72 (1): 72–80.

Roy, Cynthia B. (2000) *Interpreting as a Discourse Process*. New York: Oxford University Press.

Schegloff, Emanuel A. (2007) *Sequence Organization in Interaction: A Primer in Conversation Analysis*. Cambridge: Cambridge University Press. https://doi.org/10.1017/CBO9780511791208

Schegloff, Emanuel A., Gail Jefferson and Harvey Sacks (1977) The preference for self-correction in the organization of repair in conversation. *Language* 53 (2): 361–382. https://doi.org/10.1353/lan.1977.0041

Sidnell, Jack and Tanya Stivers (eds) (2013) *The Handbook of Conversation Analysis*. Oxford: Blackwell. https://doi.org/10.1002/9781118325001

Stivers, Tanya and Jeffrey D. Robinson (2006) A preference for progressivity in interaction. *Language in Society* 35 (3): 367–392. https://doi.org/10.1017/S0047404506060179

Valero-Garcés, Carmen (2005) Doctor–patient consultations in dyadic and triadic exchanges. *Interpreting* 7 (2): 193–210. https://doi.org/10.1075/intp.7.2.04val

Wadensjö, Cecilia (1998) *Interpreting as Interaction*. Harlow, UK: Addison Wesley Longman.

Wadensjö, Cecilia (2001) Interpreting in crisis: The interpreter's position in therapeutic encounters. In Ian Mason (ed.) *Triadic Exchanges: Studies in Dialogue Interpreting*, 71–85. Manchester: St Jerome.

Galina B. Bolden (Ph.D., UCLA) is Professor in the Department of Communication at Rutgers University. Broadly, her research examines how participants enact and negotiate their cultural identities and personal relationships in and through talk-in-interaction. She is a co-author (with Alexa Hepburn) of *Transcribing for Social Research* (2017, Sage) and co-editor (with John Heritage and Marja-Leena Sorjonen) of *Responding to Polar Questions Across Languages and Contexts* (2023, John Benjamins). Address for correspondence: Department of Communication, Rutgers University, 4 Huntington Street, New Brunswick, NJ 08901, USA. Email: gbolden@comminfo.rutgers.edu

4 Managing uncertainty in healthcare interpreter-mediated interaction: On rendering question-answer sequences

Claudio Baraldi & Laura Gavioli

4.1 The management of uncertainty in doctor–patient talk

Studies of healthcare interactions involving migrants and language interpreters have shown that interpreters coordinate participation, actively intervening as distributors and coordinators of opportunities to talk in encounters in which language barriers restrict participation (Wadensjö 1998; Mason 2006; Baraldi and Gavioli 2015), a condition which is referred to in this volume as one of communicative vulnerability. The function of 'mediation' has thus become a subject of debate in dialogue interpreting research, referring both to the dynamics of language clarification and explanation and to ways of addressing expectations which might be 'culturally' different among participants (see e.g. Angelelli 2004; Pöchhacker 2008; Baraldi and Gavioli 2015, 2017).

This paper analyses the conditions of uncertainty management in interpreter-mediated interaction in medical settings. The impossibility of direct interaction between doctors and patients without the help of a language mediator makes it necessary for interpreters to collaborate in the achievement of effective communication, thus reducing potential vulnerability. Here we look at the ways in which interpreters collaborate in accomplishing communication by rendering doctors' questions and patients' answers. We look at interpreted sequences usually occurring at the beginning of the encounters, during those phases that are labelled by Heritage and Clayman (2010) 'problem presentation' and 'history taking'.

Our analysis aims to highlight interpreters' actions which seem apt for managing uncertainty in communication effectively.

Similar to some other studies in this volume (particularly Angelelli, Wadensjö, Bolden and Twilt *et al.*), our work is based on a collection of interpreter-mediated interactions recorded during field work in collaboration with local healthcare services. In the next section we introduce the problem by means of a literature review, after which we present the data (Section 3) and then the development of the interlocutors' actions in selected data extracts (Section 4). We conclude by pointing out what it means to manage uncertainty effectively in healthcare interactions.

4.2 Literature review

The problem of uncertainty in (medical) interaction

Uncertainty in communication processes is here defined as a lack of predictability of communicative actions and of motives for acting communicatively (Gudykunst 1994; Luhmann 1994). It is an unavoidable aspect of all types of communication, and it requires some form of management. Forms of management are normally oriented to structures of the social system which provide stable expectations for action, and these expectations in turn depend on the social system involved. In Western societies for example, forms of management are expected to be oriented to pursuing right in the law system, to the democratic exercise of power in political systems and to the accomplishment of love in families (Luhmann 2012). It follows that forms of uncertainty management, oriented to the treatment of illness, will constitute characterizing features of healthcare interaction in general and interpreter-mediated healthcare interaction in particular.

By establishing forms of communication that make actions more predictable, these social structures do not provide certainty, but make uncertainty less probable in communication. Probability, as intended here, does not have a statistical meaning; rather, it indicates the stability of social systems, in that laws, politics and families are all meant to fulfil stable functions in society, and the corresponding predictability of communication processes in reference to such stability. In the healthcare system, for example, the function and form of healing may motivate patients to provide accurate information to doctors. Patients' motivation may, thus, on the basis of the primary relevance of their illness alone (Luhmann 1990), reduce uncertainty of patients' actions in medical communication.

The constitution of modern medical systems has made uncertainty improbable through well-established hierarchical relationships. Doctors manage uncertainty of patients' actions by orienting their own actions to their medical authority as experts of the field (Mishler 1984; Barry *et al.* 2001) and patients are expected to respect that medical authority, given their primary interest in healing. The role asymmetry deriving from such a hierarchical relationship can be considered a permanent feature of medical interaction (Pilnick and Dingwall 2011; see also Sarangi, this volume). However, conversation analysis (CA) has worked extensively on doctor–patient interaction (e.g. Heritage and Maynard 2006; Collins *et al.* 2007; Heritage and Clayman 2010) and has shown that patients may produce uncertainty in communication by displaying perceptions, expectations, emotions, opinions, hesitations, doubts and also resilience (e.g. Stivers 2002, 2005a, 2005b; Cohn *et al.* 2009; Paterniti *et al.* 2010; Bergen and Stivers 2013) despite doctors' traditional orientation to their authority as experts in the field.

Work in CA has also indicated, though, that rather than using their authority to account for their actions, doctors can better use their expertise to design their actions in ways which may help patients' participation (Beach and Dixson 2001; Robinson 2001; Jones and Collins 2007; Ruusuvuori 2007; Clemente *et al.* 2008; see also Bolden, this volume). Patients' active participation has been highlighted as of primary importance for successful healthcare interaction, in that it provides an interesting, reliable and 'authoritative' source of information for the doctors to make their diagnoses correctly. As such, patients' participation and involvement can be observed as part of the system's expectations.

Doctors' questions encourage patients' participation by showing attentiveness to the symptoms that prompt patients to seek medical care (problem attentiveness) and sensitivity to patients' needs (recipient design) (Heritage 2010; Heritage and Clayman 2010). In this way, doctors' questions make possible an accurate understanding of patients' symptoms and illnesses: patients' actions are treated as a resource for medical communication and uncertainty in patient actions is thus made improbable. The design of question-answer sequences then displays orientations to treat patients' responses as relevant to the objectives of the examination (Heritage and Robinson 2006; Heritage *et al.* 2007; Heritage 2010; Deppermann and Spranz-Fogasy 2011; Clemente *et al.* 2012). Question-answer sequences may thus provide for interesting material to observe the interactional management of uncertainty in medical communication. This paper investigates the ways in which these sequences are affected by the presence of an interpreter in a context that may be considered subject to communication vulnerability.

The management of uncertainty in interpreter-mediated interaction with migrant patients

Language barriers create a number of problems for the participation of migrants in interaction about their healthcare (Moss and Roberts 2005; Meeuwesen *et al.* 2007; Twilt *at al.*, this volume), resulting in silences and affecting their lexical choices and prosody (Roberts and Sarangi 2005: 637). Language barriers also create difficulties in patients' expression of emotional cues and concerns (De Maesschalck *et al.* 2011; Kale *et al.* 2011), and in shared decision making (Suurmond and Seeleman 2006). Moreover, language barriers increase the likelihood of symptoms being inadequately detected (Bischoff *et al.* 2003), of wrong diagnoses and treatments (Suurmond and Seeleman 2006) and of negative assessments by providers of the communication process (Harmsen *et al.* 2008). Such barriers thus increase uncertainty in communication, in that they (a) reduce the patients' opportunity to explain their problems and (b) impede regarding these patients as resources of relevant and authoritative medical information.

Dialogue interpreting may affect uncertainty management in different and contrasting ways. On the one hand, interpreters' mediation may support the achievement both of patients' active participation and of medical tasks, thus enhancing doctor–patient communication (Angelelli 2004; Baraldi and Gavioli 2007; Baraldi 2009; Gavioli and Baraldi 2011; Bridges *et al.* 2011; Angelelli 2012; Baraldi 2012; Gavioli 2012; Penn and Watermeyer 2012; Leanza *et al.* 2013; Baraldi and Gavioli 2015; Gavioli 2015) and improving uncertainty management in the interaction. On the other hand, though, due to the difficulty or impossibility of direct communication between doctors and patients, dialogue interpreting may introduce new forms of uncertainty. In this perspective, interpreting may not guarantee that medical communication takes place successfully, and it may instead be itself a source of trouble in communication (e.g. Cambridge 1999; Tebble 1999; Bolden 2000; Davidson 2000; Aranguri *et al.* 2006; Hsieh 2006).

Against this contradictory background, conditions of uncertainty management in interpreter-mediated communication in medical settings need further analysis. On the one side, we have data from monolingual medical interaction which suggest that doctors and patients may collaborate in the management of uncertainty by negotiating details of patients' problems and reinterpreting these as relevant and authoritative issues. On the other side, interpreters may collaborate in the achievement of effective communication by rendering questions and answers in a way that takes into account doctors' display of attention, patients' comfort and the design of doctors' search for relevant details. Insofar as patients' (as well as doctors') participation requires and depends on interpreting, medical questioning is thus the result of a triadic interaction that includes the mediator's interpreting activity as a crucial activity in uncertainty management.

In what follows, we analyse data showing how such triadic coordination takes place and its effects on uncertainty management, looking at interpreted sequences of doctors' questions and patients' answers during the phases of problem presentation and history taking. Our analysis aims to highlight actions which seem effective in gathering relevant and authoritative information from patients and that thus reduce uncertainty in communication. Effective uncertainty management is frequent in our corpus; however, it should be noted that there are also cases in which mediators' initiatives are not aligned with the aim of collecting relevant information for doctors (Angelelli, this volume).

4.3 Data and method

Our data consist of audio-recordings and transcriptions of naturally occurring interactions involving doctors, migrant patients and intercultural mediators in healthcare settings. Intercultural mediators, in ours as well as in many other Italian healthcare services, are employed for their knowledge of languages and cultures. They are not 'certified' interpreters, and they are involved in an *ad hoc* continuous training program at the institutions they work for. They are preferred over professional interpreters in that they are assumed to be more competent in dealing with the possibly different 'cultural' perspectives of healthcare providers and migrant patients. Therefore, mediators are engaged both as interpreters and as experts of cultures and intercultural communication.

The mediated interactions were recorded in two adjacent areas in northern Italy which between them host one of the highest percentages of migrant patients in the country. The data consist of approximately 300 Arabic–Italian and English–Italian interactions involving patients from North Africa (Morocco), West Africa (Ghana, Nigeria) and the Middle East. Six mediators were involved in the study (three for Arabic–Italian and three for English–Italian interactions); they were all women in their thirties, and intended to be from the same (or 'nearby') migrant communities as the patients. All data were gathered following the guidelines of the internal ethics committee of the healthcare service, which included informed consent and authorization for the use of data.

The interactions were audio-recorded and transcribed according to the conventions of conversation analysis (see Appendix), with the addition of some field notes taken by the transcribers who assisted in the collection of the data. Transcribing multiple-language conversations, particularly when a language has a non-Roman written form, raises a number of issues (see Egbert *et al.* 2016) that cannot be discussed in detail here. The decision was taken to Romanize the Arabic, for two main reasons: first, the classical Arabic written form does not always capture the diversity of spoken Arabic, and we found that speakers of different varieties read different words from our initial attempt to transcribe into Arabic script; and second, the right-to-left directionality of the Arabic script made it impossible to use alongside Italian in transcriptions, particularly as regards mixed and overlapping turns.

The method of conversation analysis highlights the ways participants make sense of their own and others' contributions. It thus seemed particularly suitable for observing the ways in which interpreters make sense of their own and the doctors' and patients' contributions by translating for them.

4.4 Analysis

The data below show four different types of sequences occurring in both the Arabic and the English datasets. These sequences are indicative of the interactional work that may be involved in the management of uncertainty in medical interpreted interaction. The sequences go from the doctor's question to the doctor's receipt of the sought detail(s) confirming that these are the wanted detail(s). As compared to monolingual doctor–patient interaction, our interpreter-mediated data show a complex interplay between doctors' design of questions and interpreter–patient sequences of responsive talk, where such design is made clear and the patients are helped to react accordingly. This interplay shows how uncertainty is produced in the interaction, and the ways in which it is managed through coordination between the doctor and the mediator.

The four types of sequences display different forms of rendition matching different interactional functions. They range from smooth turn-by-turn rendition patterns (Section 4.1) to more complex ones that include dyadic sequences between the mediator and the patient (Sections 4.2, 4.3 and 4.4). Evidence of uncertainty management activity increases in parallel with (a) the space that is allowed for the patients' participation in the interaction and (b) more complex rendition forms which involve mediator's engagement in (even longish) dyadic sequences.

Collecting details for history taking

The simplest type of sequence that follows a doctor's question includes the mediator's rendition of this question, the patient's answer and the mediator's rendition of the answer back to the doctor, as in Extracts 1 and 2 below.

Excerpt 1: (D = Doctor; M = Mediator; P = Patient)

01 D: Allora, adesso mi dovrebbe dire quando è stata l'ultima mestruazione.
Now, she should tell me when she had her last period.
02 M: Ekher regl jatak.
Last period you had.
03 P: Le seize septembre.
Sixteenth September.
04 M: Il sedici settembre.
Sixteenth September.
05 D: Okay, il sedici settembre.
Okay, sixteenth September.

In Extract 1, the doctor asks a question, the mediator renders it into Arabic, the patient answers and the mediator then renders the answer back to the doctor. Although the doctor has no mastery of the Arabic language (or French, used in turn 3), this sequence shows that uncertainty, basically deriving from the lack of direct communication between the doctor and the patient, is easily managed. What is sought for by the doctor is easily collected through the mediator's translation and rendered back to the doctor, who acknowledges receipt in turn 5.

Extract 2, below, shows a similar occurrence.

Excerpt 2

01 D: E da quanto tempo?
and for how long?
02 M: For how long?
03 P: °Eh, two weeks now°
04 M: Due settimane.
Two weeks.
(2.0)
05 D: E' la prima volta che le succede?
Is this the first time this happens to her?
06 M: Is it the first time it happen?
07 P: °Mhm, yes°
08 M: Sì.
Yes.
09 D: And the last menstruation when did it started?

Here we have a series of doctor's questions (turns 1 and 5) which are rendered in the next turn by the mediator, then answered by the patient with such answer being rendered immediately back to the doctor. In this case, there is no acknowledgment on the part of the doctor, who, after a short pause, passes to the next question. The doctor's second question (turn 5) shows that the mediator's rendition has been understood, and questioning can continue smoothly. A third doctor's question is asked in turn 9, showing that the questioning sequence is still going on smoothly (and that the doctor is learning some English, since she dares asking using the patient's language).

Working on the dynamics of the presentation of patients' problems in monolingual medical interactions, Heritage and Robinson (2006) distinguish several types of doctors' questions. Some are general, open-ended questions, like 'how are you?' questions, which project expectations for unconditioned patients' responses. Others, like symptom confirmations, glosses or history-taking questions, instead project sharply constrained closed-ended responses, such as 'yes-no' answers, a choice from options or the provision of details, e.g. dates, age, names and the like (Heritage and Robinson 2006: 97). The doctors' questions we have seen above are of the latter type. Insofar as they seek specific information regarding the medical history of the patient, these questions are designed as 'inquiring' and focused (Robinson 2001). In interpreted interaction, doctors' questions are responded to first and foremost by the mediators, who interpret the doctors' design and re-design their renditions. Such a re-designing operation normally makes the focus of the doctors' questions clear and precise, reduces it to the core and gets directly to the answer sought for – which is in its turn rendered immediately and quickly to the doctor.

This design of doctors' questions is effective in managing uncertainty in that it provides constraints which stabilize both mediators' interpreting and patients' difficulties of participation. Being closed-ended, these questions diminish the range of interpretability sharply, thus favouring effective turn-by-turn close rendition of speakers' utterances.

The presentation of patients' problems: Inviting patients' expansions

While 'how are you?' questions are rare in our data, other types of general questions are quite common. This is the case with general inquiry questions, such as 'what's your problem?'. As noted by Heritage and Robinson (2006), these questions are designed to invite the presentation of patients' problems and allow patients to talk about their concerns in their own terms, describing symptoms or providing more extensive narratives of their diseases. In monolingual talk, these patients' presentations are responded to by the doctors, who either guide the patients to say more, or ask for confirmation and check details.

In our data, feedback to the patients' presentations of symptoms is normally provided by the mediator, who thus engages in dyadic talk with patients. As shown in the literature on dialogue interpreting (e.g. Wadensjö 1998; Mason 2006), dyadic sequences in interpreter-mediated interactions are quite common and have been described as functional to establishing reciprocity in talk where linguistic barriers do not allow participants to provide direct feedback to each other (Davidson 2002).

In the data we will see in this and the following sections, dyadic sequences with different functions are negotiated by participants in the interaction. Extracts 3 and 4 below show two cases, both following a doctor's general inquiry question. In the first extract, the patient tells about some worrying heart symptoms; in the second, we have a report of a urination problem. In both cases, the patient's telling is reacted to by the mediator.

Excerpt 3

01 D: Okay dimmi adesso.
Okay please tell me now.

02 M: So what's your problem now? (??)
03 P: My heart is worrying me, my heart.
04 M: How is it worrying you?
05 P: Ehm: my heart is- ((showing with hand gesture))
06 M: Beating faster?
07 P: Yes, yes, beat fast (.) fast fast.
08 M: Or you feel pain?
09 P: Ye-yes, I feel pain. (As straight work)
10 M: It beats faster?
11 P: Yes.
12 M: Eh:: ha il cuore che batte forte. Ha anche dolore (.) dice.
Eh:: her heart beats fast. She has got pain too
13 D: Da quanto?
How long?

Here, following the interpreted invitation by the doctor ('what's your problem?'), the patient presents the reason for his worry ('my heart is worrying me'). The mediator reacts with three subsequent questions, seeking more specific details: first, asking what precisely worries the patient about his heart ('how is it worrying you?', turn 4); second, attempting to interpret his gesture (turn 5); and third, suggesting other possible symptoms (turn 8). The details, thus collected, are eventually rendered to the doctor in turn 12; the doctor shifts to her next question in turn 13.

While the mediator's questions seemingly substitute the doctor's, there are two important differences. First, the mediator's questions focus on possible expansions of details previously given by the patient: in this sense, although the questions dig for more and more precise details, they are not 'new' history-taking questions. Second, and possibly more significantly, the mediator does not provide any type of acknowledgment ('mhm' or 'okay') about the relevance of the details provided by the patient, and only renders them back to the doctor. It is the doctor who confirms the relevance of the details by asking new, relevant questions.

Extract 4 provides another example of a general inquiry question, inviting the patient's problem presentation. Interestingly, the doctor's question includes the mediator as an interlocutor ('Please tell <u>us</u>', rather than 'tell <u>me</u>').

Excerpt 4

01 D: Dicci pure.
Please, tell us. ((your story))
02 M: Ashnu lmuskil?
What's the problem?

03 P: Baqi fiha hadaq li kan bul u kat jini lbula fisa' u ltht walla ki hbat minni lma.
I keep having ((the problem)) that when I have to pee it comes all of a sudden and water starts to leak.
04 M: Nti hkiti ma'ahum min kbal?
Did you speak with them before?
05 P: Mmh.
06 M: Hkiti 'al mushkil hada kbal?
Did you tell somebody ((doctors)) about this problem
07 P: Ah.
Yes.
08 M: Dice che è qua per il problema dell'urinare diciamo.
She says that the problem she has is let's say to urinate.
09 D: Mmh?
10 M: Nel senso che le dà fastidio.
In the sense that it is bothering her.
11 M: Ya'ni nti lwaqt li tbul thib tirja' fisa'.
That is when you need to pee, you immediately need it again.
12 P: Ah, fisa' u kan lqa lkharka diali fiha shihaja safra ma bkatsh kat 'jabni.
Yes, immediately, and I find something yellow in my underpants, which I don't like.
13 M: Ha delle perdite gialle (.) e in più il problema dell'[urina.
She has a yellow discharge plus the problem of [urine.
14 P: [Ualakin bla riha.
However, without smell.
15 M: Sì, con l'urina ha l'istinto o la voglia ancora di urinare [nuovo direttamente.
Yes, with urine she feels like she has the instinct or desire to urinate [again and again, straightaway.
16 D: [nuovo.
Again and again.
17 D: questo disturbo da quanto ce l'ha?
When did this problem start?

As in Extract 3, the doctor's question is rendered with a routine inquiry question form: 'what's the problem?'. The patient's narrative starts at turn 3, where she mentions a problem that has lasted for a while; the mediator reacts by asking if the problem is known to the doctors, and the patient confirms. This prompts the mediator to render the first part of the story to the doctor (turn 8). The doctor's reaction though shows that the problem is new to her, so the mediator gets back to the patient to collect more details. In turn 11, she checks her understanding of the problem with the patient. In turn 12, the patient confirms that the mediator's understanding of the problem is correct and adds more details, at which point the complete story is rendered to the doctor, who finally acknowledges that this is recognizable, relevant and authoritative information.

In Extracts 3 and 4 the doctor's general inquiry questions prompt the patients to tell their problems. In both cases, the patients are helped by the mediators to expand their problem presentation and include more details on recognizably relevant symptoms. The mediator's talk with the patient may produce uncertainty in communication in two ways: (1) by leaving the doctor temporarily with no access to what the patient says; and (2) by the risk that it is the mediator, not the doctor, who negotiates the relevance of the details given in the patient's problem presentation, possibly mismanaging their medical relevance. Forms of uncertainty management can, however, be observed in the mediators' coordinating work: (1) their questions focus on the expansion of details previously presented by the patients, from more general to more specific; and (2) the mediators never acknowledge the information obtained as relevant to the examination – when the collection of details is held to be 'enough', it is rendered to the doctor and it is the doctor who provides acknowledgments and moves the interaction on.

The doctors also contribute in the management of uncertainty in these interactions, by authorizing the mediators' activity in at least three ways: (1) by acknowledging the details collected by the interpreters as worthy of medical attention; (2) by using we-forms in their general inquiry questions ('tell us', meaning 'me and the mediator' – see Extract 4, turn 1), which suggests that the mediator is competent in helping the doctor collect relevant information; and (3) by encouraging the mediators to collect more details. In Extract 4, for instance, after the mediator's rendition of the first part of the patient's expansion, the doctor's contribution ('mhm', turn 9) works both as a partial acknowledgment and as a continuer of the mediator's activity.

While engagement into mediator–patient dyadic sequences may lower the doctor's control of the interaction (by leaving the doctor aside), they may conversely consolidate their control over the interactional activity, in that the doctor authorizes the mediator to engage in dyadic sequences and acknowledges such sequences as functional to continuing medical inquiries and to starting the history-taking phase. The doctor's medical authority is thus exercised by enhancing the communicative expertise of the mediator in collecting and rendering patients' tellings on their behalf.

Patients' replies to history-taking questions

As interactions are constructed with contributions from all the participants (Angelelli, this volume), there are occurrences where the particular doctor's question designs are not (immediately) taken up in the following talk. This is the case when focused history-taking questions, rendered by the mediator in the patient's language, are followed by more a general patient's narrative. In these cases, interactional uncertainty is managed in order to be conducive to the detail sought by the doctor.

In Extract 5 it is the mediator who engages in dyadic talk with the patient and contributes to the accomplishment of his answer, while in Extract 6 it is the doctor who, after a lengthy story by the patient provided with the help of the mediator, brings the focus back to the detail she was looking for.

Excerpt 5

1 D: Ha avuto dei rapporti non protetti?
Did he have unprotected sexual intercourse?
2 M: 'milti - (..) ha ullaha eh bi al'arabya (.) 'alaka jinsia min 'eir l'ajil ṯibbi, min 'eir l'ajil ṯibbi?
Did you do – (..) as you say in Arabic (.) sexual intercourse out of medical protection, out of medical protection
3 P: Ana thalatha sinin hina -
I have been here for three years -
4 M: Ma 'andaksh shi 'alaka jinsia?
Don't you have sexual intercourse?
5 P: Lâ lâ lâ.
No no no.
6 M: E' da tre anni che non fa niente.
He has not been doing anything for three years.
7 D: Oltre il sangue, diciamo, cola anche altro materiale oppure solo quando eiacula che ha sangue?
Besides blood, I mean, is there any other material leaking or is it only during ejaculation that he has blood?

In Extract 5, the doctor's question in turn 1 ('did he have unprotected sexual intercourse') seeks for a specific yes/no answer. After the mediator's rendition in Arabic, the patient's answer is quite general 'I have been here for three years'). The mediator then asks the patient explicitly if his answer means that he had no sexual intercourse for three years. The patient's confirmation (in turn 5) is rendered to the doctor (in turn 6), who moves on to the next question (in turn 7).

In Extract 6, instead, the doctor's focused, history-taking question ('when were the children born?') follows a long conversation where the doctor and the mediator are trying to understand a very complicated patient's history (data not shown).

Excerpt 6

1 D: Gemellare. E quando ha – (.) sono nati i bambini?
Twins. And when she has – (.) were the children born?

2 M: Eh – le jumeaux waslu, ya'ni, walattum'adi ya'ni –
Eh – the twins arrived, I mean, did you give birth to them normally, I mean –

3 P: Khit tbeba shahar laual,'tatni traitement shhar laual,'tatni traitement.
I took the first month, the doctor gave me the treatment, the first month she gave me the treatment

4 M: Ya'ni bditi mn laual.
I mean you started from the beginning.

5 P: Ah, mn shhar laual.
Yes, from the first month.

6 M: Okay, con la seconda gravidanza –
Okay, with the first pregnancy –

7 P: No.

8 M: Mmh.

9 P: Kat 'barlia la pression mziana, kulla shhar kan dir l'ecografie, chac mois kan dir l'ecografie (.)'ada mziana (..) shahar sab' (?) mn ba'd 15 yum dkhalt 'autani, dkhalt 'autani qabluni.
She measured well my blood pressure, each month I did the ultrasound scan, each month I did the ultrasound scan (.) I did well (.) did well (..) the seventh month (?) after fifteen days I went again ((in the hospital)), *I went again and they accepted me.*

10 M: Allora, con la seconda gravidanza ha detto che la pressione è alzata dall'inizio e ha cominciato a fare una terapia con il medico (.) poi: eh (.) ad un certo punto il settimo mese è stata ricoverata in ospedale perché aveva la pressione altissima eh (.) a trentatré settimane hanno visto che i bambini (.) uno dei bambini non ce la faceva, era già debole e hanno deciso di fargli il cesareo (..) operare tutte due, praticamente li hanno tirati via.
So, with the second pregnancy she said that the pressure increased from the beginning and she started a therapy with the doctor (.) then: eh (.) at a certain point in the seventh month she was hospitalized because she had a very high blood pressure eh (.) at thirty-three weeks they saw that the children (.) one of the children couldn't do it, he was already weak and they decided to do a caesarean section (.) do a surgery for both, in practice they took them away.

11 D: Quindi, in che anno sempre?
So, which year this too?

The mediator's rendition (turn 2) is apparently mismatched: while the doctor wanted to know whether the pregnancy with twins, which had been mentioned by the patient, had come to term successfully (rather than ending in miscarriage or stillbirth), the mediator focuses on whether the birth took place normally. In her reply, starting in turn 3, the patient tells a story revealing that she had very high blood pressure during her pregnancy, which led the doctors to perform a caesarean section. This story is rendered by the mediator in turns 6 and 10. The doctor's follow-up question in turn 11 acknowledges the relevance of the patient's story for the medical examination and also insists on the doctor's previously requested point: when did all this take place? By this question, the doctor acknowledges the relevance of the work of the mediator, which went rather beyond the doctor's initial question, and brings the interaction back to the focus of that initial question.

In summary, in Extracts 5 and 6 the patients' answers deviate from the doctors' projected trajectories. In both cases, the answer is put 'back on track' – by the mediator in Extract 5 and by the doctor in Extract 6. In both cases, the doctor acknowledges the relevance of the work of the mediator and includes the received information in their next question. It is interesting to observe that while the mediator and the doctor cooperate in the accomplishment of sequences where the patients' answers eventually match the doctor's questions, the actual patients' answers are quite free and include a number of possibly (but not necessarily) relevant details. In both making sense of the patient's 'non-conforming' answer explicit in Extract 5 and in acknowledging the relevance of the patient's story in Extract 6, their contributions are enhanced and appreciated as relevant and enriching for the current interactional goals. In other words, interactional uncertainty which may be produced by patients' non-conforming answers is made stable by treating such answers as relevant to the communication system.

Ambiguous patient answers

The last pattern considered here involves cases where a doctor's focused, history-taking question, rendered by the mediator closely and immediately in the following turn, is answered by the patient in a way that is treated in the interaction as problematic. We have called these answers 'ambiguous' because while they are definitely relevant answers to the doctor's questions and provide the requested details, they may have ambiguous implications for the patient's illness. In these cases uncertainty is managed by the doctor and the mediator cooperating to solve the ambiguity and deal with possible implications deriving from the patient's answer. Extracts 7 and 8 provide two examples of this.

Excerpt 7

1 D: Ultima mestruazione quando è stata?
Last menstruation when was it?
2 M: Akhir marra jatk fiha l 'ada shahriya?
Last time you had your period?
3 P: Rab'awa'ishrin (.) f sh'har juj.
Twenty-fourth (.) in the month of February.
(02)
4 M: F sh'har juj?
In February?
5 P: Ah, rab'awa'ishrin (.) f sh'har juj.
Yes, twenty-fourth of February.
6 M: F sh'har- f had sh'har ma jatksh?
In the month- in this month you didn't have it?
7 P: Majatnish, yallah jatni, ghlt lik dart liya retard tis' ayyam.
I didn't have, I have just had it, I told you I had a nine-day delay.
8 M: Yallah jatk?
You've just had it?
9 P: Ah.
Yes.
10 M: Imta jatk?
When did you have it?
11 P: Jatni:: el bareh.
I had it yesterday.
12 M: Ehm, ya'ni les regles tsamma dyal l bareh mush-
Ehm so yesterday menstruation don't-
13 P: Ah, ghlt dyal bareh, mashi lli ghlt dak sh'har.
as I said yesterday, not that from last month.
14 M: Eh, no, akher marra. ma'natha nti daba haid?
Well no, last time. So you're having your period now?
15 P: Ah.
Yes.
16 M: Allora, attualmente è mestruata. (.) Le sono venute ieri.
Well, she's having her period now (.) It came yesterday.
17 D: ah! Allora bisogna che torni.
Ah! So she has to come back.

In Extract 7, a doctor's routine, history-taking question (last menstruation date, turn 1) is rendered closely by the mediator in turn 2. The patient's answer (twenty-fourth February, turn 5) provides the relevant detail, the menstruation date, but a date which is longer than a month before. The ambiguity thus concerns the possibility that the patient either (a) misunderstood the question or (b) has a significant menstrual delay, which, as such, needs to be reported to the doctor. In turn 4, then, the mediator starts a clarification sequence to solve this ambiguity. In turns 7–15, it is made clear by the patient that 24 February is the date of her previous menstruation and that she is currently having her period after a delay of nine days. The mediator's rendition in turn 16 restores interactional management on the part of the doctor.

In this extract, then, the ambiguity of the patient's answer is managed and solved by the interpreter, who engages in a dyadic sequence with the patient in order to clarify the meaning of the provided detail. The doctor does not interrupt the sequence and reacts to the mediator's rendition, treating the provided information as worthy of medical attention (if the patient is having her period, she cannot take the test today).

Extract 8 opens in a very similar way.

Excerpt 8

01 D: lei prende de:l contraccettivo?
Does she take any contraceptive?
02 M: are you taking the pills?
03 P: no I: don't take it never gimme:: I don't want really taking this.
04 M: Really.
05 P: Yes.
06 M: do you want pregnancy now.
07 P: I don't want pregnancy what I(?) I don't have a boyfriend that(?)for me.
08 M: ma:
09 P: aw I don't want really take it.
10 M: non ha un ragazzo quindi non serve più la pillola (.) quindi non ha ragazzo con cui: eh utilizza: mmm che fa senza:: l'uso dei condom.
she doesn't have a boyfriend so pills are not necessary (.) so she doesn't have a boyfriend with who:m eh she use:s mm she does without::t using condoms.

The doctor's history-taking question (turn 1) is rendered closely and immediately by the mediator in the following turn (turn 2). The ambiguous answer by the patient comes in turn 3, where she answers 'no' and adds that she does not want to take contraceptive pills. Since promoting protected sex is one of the goals of this healthcare service, the mediator attributes this answer a medical relevance and opens a dyadic sequence with the patient to clarify the reason why she does not want to take oral contraception, possibly interpreting such patient's explanation as potentially relevant for the doctor. In turns 4–9, it is clarified that the patient does not have a boyfriend, and so she does not want to take pills. The mediator's rendition in turn 10 brings the interactional management back to the doctor, who explores the patient's situation further and suggests an alternative contraception method. It is probably worth clarifying that medical concern for contraception is particularly high in this clinic, which often assists women engaged in sex work.

In summary, Extracts 7 and 8 show two cases where a patient's ambiguous answer needs some work before the sequence reaches a conclusion. Clarification sequences are opened by the mediators to solve the ambiguity and render relevant details to the doctor. Uncertainty management here focuses on the actual significance of the patients' answers for their examination and their illnesses. The patient's contribution is in both cases treated as relevant, and its meaning explored to check whether more details of medical relevance can be given to the doctor. In both cases, the interaction is put back on track: in Extract 7, by the mediator through solving the misunderstanding, and in Extract 8 by the doctor, who accepts the patient's position and suggests an alternative contraceptive method.

4.5 Discussion and conclusion

Our analysis suggests that in interpreted encounters, as in monolingual interaction, the enhancement of patients' contribution to healthcare communication involves mitigation of doctors' orientation to medical authority. Mediators' authority in interpreting is an additional resource for medical communication, which has relevant effects in balancing doctors' and patients' contributions. As in monolingual interaction, doctors can use their expertise in designing their contributions for their patients and showing attentiveness to their patients' telling. In interpreter-mediated communication, this work can effectively be done through the mediator's cooperation: on a basic level, mediators engage in talk with the patients and collect details which may be relevant for medical examination and diagnosis.

Mediators, however, do much more than collect details: using expertise acquired during previous experiences of mediation in this or similar settings, they help doctors' question designs get through; they enhance attention for 'un-matching' patient answers; and they explore and eventually accomplish their relevance in the interaction. These aspects of mediators' action are shown in our data, in those cases where patients' information cannot be treated, easily and directly, as relevant for the doctor.

On the first point, of question design, the extracts show this in three contexts. The first is that of general inquiry sequences launched by doctors: as research on monolingual interaction shows, patients' first answers can be incomplete and in need of further investigation, so possible uncertainty deriving from patients' telling is likely to occur. In our data, it is the mediator, not the doctor, who manages uncertain developments of patients' talk, in dyadic interaction with the patients, and renders deliverable information to the doctors. The second, possibly similar context is that of patients' extended answers to focused doctors' questions. In our data, as with monolingual interaction, these lengthy answers do not provide straightforward replies to doctors' requests, so some work needs to be done to negotiate their relevance. Here too, it is the mediator who manages the relevance of the patients' expansions. The third context is that of ambiguous patients' answers. In our data, this is probably where uncertainty is more evident. Insofar as, in the management of these answers, mediators use some (basic) medical knowledge, this creates a risk for doctor/mediator role-overlapping.

In each case, uncertainty management is conducted in close collaboration by the mediator and the doctor. While the mediator contingently separates the doctor and the patient and may thus be held to assume the role of 'co-diagnostician' (Hsieh 2006), our data show two types of possibly interesting dynamics: those which enhance the patients' contributions and make them 'valuable' in the interaction, and those by which the mediators decline assuming the role of (co-)diagnostician and align as 'interpreters'. In the former case, the mediators in our data guide the patients to appreciate the sense of the doctors' questions; they also solicit more details from the patients, solve possible misunderstandings and improve the communicative relevance of the patients' narratives to achieve correct understanding of the patients' conditions. In the latter instance, while the mediators work to clarify the details provided by the patients and their possible relevance in medical talk, they systematically decline the task of evaluating the actual relevance of the information. Through their renditions of the gathered details to the doctor, the mediators put the coordination of the interaction back in the hands of the doctor, who is ultimately responsible for acknowledging the relevance of the details and moving the interaction on.

Research shows that, in monolingual interaction, migrant patients either do not participate or participate with severe linguistic difficulties. In our interpreted-mediated data, one feature which can probably be appreciated is that although they produce incomplete, apparently irrelevant or ambiguous contributions, the migrant patients participate actively. Such active participation needs to be managed through translation, since doctors cannot intervene directly in a language they do not speak. This requires collaboration with mediators, who are those who have access to the patients' language; but when patients' contributions show uncertainty, immediate rendering may not be enough for doctors to be able to manage the system stability. Mediators thus act autonomously in dyadic sequences with patients. Patient participation enhancement may produce uncertainty, as it requires more complex interactional work by mediators, but it gives mediators the opportunity to act on uncertainty by taking patients' problems in their hands. In this way, patients' problems and issues can be passed over to doctors who, at this point, are in a position to acknowledge the information and reprise interactional coordination medically.

In conclusion, mediated interpreting works by increasing uncertainty of the 'ordered' medical interaction, both reducing doctors' authority and enhancing patients' expansions. Paradoxically, though, an increase in uncertainty is what enhances uncertainty management and then the actual possibility of mediators (or interpreters) to balance conditions of communicative vulnerability.

Appendix: Transcription conventions

The conventions used here are based on Psathas and Anderson (1990).

(.)	barely noticeable pause
(n)	noticeable, timed pause (n = length in seconds)
text [text	overlapping talk.] indicates end of
[text	overlap (when audible)
tex-	syllable cut short
te:xt	lengthening of previous sound or syllable
(text)	unclear audio or tentative description (due to unclear audio)
(?)	untranscribable audio
=	text latched to the preceding turn in transcript

text	stressed syllable or word
TEXT	high volume
°text°	low volume
.,?!	punctuation provides a guide to intonation, when intonation is unclear, no punctuation is provided
((sneezes))	non-verbal activity or transcriber's comments
testo text	intra-turn translation in italics

References

Angelelli, Claudia V. (2004) *Medical Interpreting and Cross-Cultural Communication*. Cambridge: Cambridge University Press. https://doi.org/10.1017/CBO9780511486616

Angelelli, Claudia V. (2012) Challenges in interpreters' coordination of the construction of pain. In Claudio Baraldi and Laura Gavioli (eds) *Coordinating Participation in Dialogue Interpreting*, 251–268. Amsterdam: John Benjamins. https://doi.org/10.1075/btl.102.11ang

Aranguri, Cesar, Brad Davidson and Robert Ramirez (2006) Patterns of communication through interpreters: A detailed sociolinguistic analysis. *Journal of General Internal Medicine* 21 (6): 623–629. https://doi.org/10.1111/j.1525-1497.2006.00451.x

Baraldi, Claudio (2009) Forms of mediation. The case of interpreter-mediated interactions in medical systems. *Language and Intercultural Communication* 9 (2): 120–137. https://doi.org/10.1080/14708470802588393

Baraldi, Claudio (2012) Interpreting as dialogic mediation: The relevance of expansions. In Claudio Baraldi and Laura Gavioli (eds) *Coordinating Participation in Dialogue Interpreting*, 297–326. Amsterdam: John Benjamins. https://doi.org/10.1075/btl.102.13bar

Baraldi, Claudio and Laura Gavioli (2007) Dialogue interpreting as intercultural mediation: An analysis in healthcare multicultural settings. In Marion Grein and Edda Weigand (eds) *Dialogue and Culture*, 155–175. Amsterdam: John Benjamins. https://doi.org/10.1075/ds.1.12bar

Baraldi, Claudio and Laura Gavioli (2012) Understanding coordination in interpreter-mediated interaction. In Claudio Baraldi and Laura Gavioli (eds) *Coordinating Participation in Dialogue Interpreting*, 1–21. Amsterdam: John Benjamins. https://doi.org/10.1075/btl.102.01intro

Baraldi, Claudio and Laura Gavioli (2015) On professional and non-professional interpreting: The case of intercultural mediators. *European Journal of Applied Linguistics* 4 (1): 33–55. https://doi.org/10.1515/eujal-2015-0026

Baraldi, Claudio and Laura Gavioli (2017) Intercultural mediation and '(non)professional' interpreting in Italian healthcare institutions. In Rachele Antonini, Letizia Cirillo, Linda Rossato and Ira Torresi (eds) *Non-Professional Interpreting and Translation: State of the Art and Future of an Emerging Field of Research*, 83–106. Amsterdam: John Benjamins. https://doi.org/10.1075/btl.129.05bar

Barry, Christine A., Fiona A. Stevenson, Nicky Britten, Nick Barber and Colin P. Bradley (2001) Giving voice to the lifeworld: More human, more effective medical care? A qualitative study of doctor-patient communication in general practice. *Social Science & Medicine* 53 (4): 487–505. https://doi.org/10.1016/S0277-9536(00)00351-8

Beach, Wayne A. and Christie M. Dixson (2001) Revealing moments: Formulating understandings of adverse experiences in a health appraisal interview. *Social Science & Medicine* 52 (1): 25–44. https://doi.org/10.1016/S0277-9536(00)00118-0

Bergen, Clara and Tanya Stivers (2013) Patient disclosure of medical misdeeds. *Journal of Health and Social Behavior* 54 (2): 221–240. https://doi.org/10.1177/0022146513487379

Bischoff, Alexander, Patrick A. Bovier, Rrustemi Isah, Gariazzo Françoise, Eytan Ariel and Louis Loutan (2003) Language barriers between nurses and asylum seekers: Their impact on symptom reporting and referral. *Social Science & Medicine* 57 (3): 503–512. https://doi.org/10.1016/S0277-9536(02)00376-3

Bolden, Galina B. (2000) Toward understanding practices of medical interpreting: Interpreters' involvement in history taking. *Discourse Studies* 2 (4): 387–419. https://doi.org/10.1177/1461445600002004001

Bridges, Susan M., Cynthia Yiu and Colman McGrath (2011) Multilingual interactions in clinical dental education: A focus on mediated interpreting. *Communication & Medicine* 8 (3): 197–210. https://doi.org/10.1558/cam.v8i3.197

Cambridge, Jan (1999) Information loss in bilingual medical interviews through an untrained interpreter. *The Translator* 5 (2): 201–219. https://doi.org/10.1080/13556509.1999.10799041

Clemente, Ignasi, John Heritage, Marcia L. Meldrum, Jennie C. I. Tsao and Lonnie K. Zeltzer (2012) Preserving the child as a respondent: Initiating patient-centered interviews in a US outpatient tertiary care pediatric pain clinic. *Communication & Medicine* 9 (3): 203–213. https://doi.org/10.1558/cam.v9i3.203

Clemente, Ignasi, Seung-Hee Lee and John Heritage (2008) Children in chronic pain: Promoting paediatric patients' symptom accounts in tertiary care. *Social Science & Medicine* 66 (6): 1418–1428. https://doi.org/10.1016/j.socscimed.2007.11.015

Cohn, Ellen S., Dharma E. Cortes, Julie M. Hook, Leanne S. Yinusa-Nyahkoon, Jeffrey L. Solomon and Barbara Bokhour (2009) A narrative of resistance: Presentation of self when parenting with children with asthma. *Communication & Medicine* 6 (1): 27–37. https://doi.org/10.1558/cam.v6i1.27

Collins, Sarah, Nicky Britten, Johanna Ruusuvuori and Andrew Thompson (eds) (2007) *Patient Participation in Health Care Consultations: Qualitative Perspectives.* Milton Keynes: Open University Press.

Davidson, Brad (2000) The interpreter as institutional gatekeeper: The social-linguistic role of interpreters in Spanish-English medical discourse. *Journal of Sociolinguistics* 4 (3): 379–405. https://doi.org/10.1111/1467-9481.00121

Davidson, Brad (2002) A model for the construction of conversational common ground in interpreted discourse. *Journal of Pragmatics* 34 (9): 1273–1300. https://doi.org/10.1016/S0378-2166(02)00025-5

De Maesschalck, Stéphanie, Myriam Deveugele and Sara Willems (2011) Language, culture and emotions: Exploring ethnic minority patients' emotional expressions in primary healthcare consultations. *Patient Education and Counseling* 84 (3): 406–412. https://doi.org/10.1016/j.pec.2011.04.021

Deppermann, Arnulf and Thomas Spranz-Fogasy (2011) Doctors' questions as displays of understanding. *Communication & Medicine* 8 (2): 111–122. https://doi.org/10.1558/cam.v8i2.111

Egbert, Maria, Mamiko Yufu and Fumiya Hirataka (2016) An investigation of how 100 articles in the Journal of Pragmatics treat transcripts of English and non-English languages. *Journal of Pragmatics* 94: 98–111. https://doi.org/10.1016/j.pragma.2016.01.010

Gavioli, Laura (2012) Minimal responses in interpreter-mediated medical talk. In Claudio Baraldi and Laura Gavioli (eds) *Coordinating Participation in Dialogue Interpreting,* 201–228. Amsterdam: John Benjamins. https://doi.org/10.1075/btl.102.09gav

Gavioli, Laura (2015) On the distribution of responsibilities in treating critical issues in interpreter-mediated medical consultations: The case of 'le spieghi(amo)'. *Journal of Pragmatics* 76: 159–180. https://doi.org/10.1016/j.pragma.2014.12.001

Gavioli, Laura and Claudio Baraldi (2011) Interpreter-mediated interaction in healthcare and legal settings: Talk organization, context and the achievement of intercultural communication. *Interpreting* 13 (2): 205–233. https://doi.org/10.1075/intp.13.2.03gav

Gudykunst, William B. (1994) *Bridging Differences: Effective Intergroup Communication*. Thousand Oaks, CA: Sage.

Harmsen, J. A. M. [Hans], Roos M. D. Bernsen, Marc A. Bruijnzeels and Ludwien Meeuwesen (2008) Patients' evaluation of quality of care in general practice: What are the cultural and linguistic barriers? *Patient Education and Counseling* 72 (1): 155–162. https://doi.org/10.1016/j.pec.2008.03.018

Heritage, John (2010) Questioning in medicine. In Alice Freed and Susan Ehrlich (eds) *'Why Do You Ask?': The Function of Questions in Institutional Discourse*, 42–68. New York: Oxford University Press.

Heritage, John and Steven Clayman (2010) 2010. *Talk in Action: Interactions, Identities, and Institutions*. Chichester, UK: Wiley-Blackwell. https://doi.org/10.1002/9781444318135

Heritage, John and Douglas W. Maynard (eds) (2006) *Communication in Medical Care: Interactions between Primary Care Physicians and Patients*. Cambridge: Cambridge University Press. https://doi.org/10.1017/CBO9780511607172

Heritage, John and Jeffrey D. Robinson (2006) The structure of patients' presenting concerns: Physicians' opening questions. *Health Communication* 19 (2): 89–102. https://doi.org/10.1207/s15327027hc1902_1

Heritage, John, Jeffrey D. Robinson, Marc N. Elliott, Megan Beckett and Michael Wilkes (2007) Reducing patients' unmet concerns in primary care: The difference one world can make. *Journal of General Internal Medicine* 22 (10): 1429–1433. https://doi.org/10.1007/s11606-007-0279-0

Hsieh, Elaine (2006) Interpreters as co-diagnosticians: Overlapping roles and services between providers and interpreters. *Social Science & Medicine* 64 (4): 924–937. https://doi.org/10.1016/j.socscimed.2006.10.015

Jones, Aled and Sarah Collins (2007) Nursing assessments and other tasks. Influences on participation in interactions between patients and nurses. In Sarah Collins, Nicky Britten, Johanna Ruusuvuori and Andrew Thompson (eds) *Patient Participation in Health Care Consultations: Qualitative Perspectives*, 143–163. Milton Keynes: Open University Press.

Kale, Kale, Arnstein Finset, Hanne-Lise Eikeland and Pål Gulbrandsen (2011) Emotional cues and concerns in hospital encounters with non-Western immigrants as compared with Norwegians: An exploratory study. *Patient Education and Counseling* 84 (3): 325–331. https://doi.org/10.1016/j.pec.2011.05.009

Leanza, Yvan, Isabelle Boivin and Ellen Rosenberg (2013) The patient's lifeworld: Building meaningful clinical encounters between patients, physicians and interpreters. *Communication & Medicine* 10 (1): 13–25. https://doi.org/10.1558/cam.v10i1.13

Luhmann, Niklas (1990) Der medizinische code. In Niklas Luhmann *Soziolgische Aufklärung 5*, 183–195. Opladen, Germany: Westdeutscher Verlag. https://doi.org/10.1007/978-3-322-97005-3_8

Luhmann, Niklas (1994) *Social Systems*. Stanford, CA: Stanford University Press.

Luhmann, Niklas (2012) *Theory of Society, Volume 1*. Stanford, CA: Stanford University Press.

Mason, Ian (2006) On mutual accessibility of contextual assumptions in dialogue interpreting. *Journal of Pragmatics* 38 (3): 359–373. https://doi.org/10.1016/j.pragma.2005.06.022

Meeuwesen, Ludwien, Fred Tromp, Barbara C. Schouten and J. A. M. [Hans] Harmsen (2007) Cultural differences in managing information during medical interaction: How does the physician get a clue? *Patient Education and Counseling* 67 (2): 183–190. https://doi.org/10.1016/j.pec.2007.03.013

Mishler, Elliot G. (1984) *The Discourse of Medicine: The Dialectics of Medical Interviews*. Norwood, NJ: Ablex.

Moss, Becky and Celia Roberts (2005) Explanations, explanations, explanations: How do patients with limited English construct narrative accounts in multi-lingual, multi-ethnic settings, and how can GPs interpret them? *Family Practice* 22 (4): 412–418. https://doi.org/10.1093/fampra/cmi037

Paterniti, Debora A., Tonya L. Fancher, Camille S. Cipri, Stefan Timmermans, John Heritage and Richard L. Kravitz (2010) Getting to 'no': Strategies primary care physicians use to deny patient requests. *Archives of Internal Medicine* 170 (4): 381–388. https://doi.org/10.1001/archinternmed.2009.533

Penn, Claire and Jennifer Watermeyer (2012) Cultural brokerage and overcoming communication barriers: A case study for aphasia. In Claudio Baraldi and Laura Gavioli (eds) *Coordinating Participation in Dialogue Interpreting*, 269–296. Amsterdam: John Benjamins. https://doi.org/10.1075/btl.102.12pen

Pilnick, Alison and Robert Dingwall (2011) On the remarkable persistence of asymmetry in doctor/patient interaction: A critical review. *Social Science & Medicine* 72 (8): 1374–1382. https://doi.org/10.1016/j.socscimed.2011.02.033

Pöchhacker, Franz (2008) Interpreting as mediation. In Carmen Valero-Garcés and Anne Martin (eds) *Crossing Borders in Community Interpreting: Definitions and Dilemmas*, 9–26. Amsterdam: John Benjamins. https://doi.org/10.1075/btl.76.02poc

Psathas George and Timothy Anderson (1990) The practices of transcription in conversation analysis. *Semiotica* 78 (1–2): 75–99. https://doi.org/10.1515/semi.1990.78.1-2.75

Roberts, Celia and Srikant Sarangi (2005) Theme-oriented discourse analysis of medical encounters. *Medical Education* 39 (6): 632–640. https://doi.org/10.1111/j.1365-2929.2005.02171.x

Robinson, Jeffrey D. (2001) Closing medical encounters: Two physician practices and their implications for the expression of patients' unstated concerns. *Social Science & Medicine* 53 (5): 639–656. https://doi.org/10.1016/S0277-9536(00)00366-X

Ruusuvuori, Johanna (2007) Managing affect: Integration of empathy and problem-solving in health care encounters. *Discourse Studies* 9 (5): 597–622. https://doi.org/10.1177/1461445607081269

Stivers, Tanya (2002) Presenting the problem in paediatric encounters: 'Symptoms only' versus 'candidate diagnosis' presentations. *Health Communication* 14 (3): 299–338. https://doi.org/10.1207/S15327027HC1403_2

Stivers, Tanya (2005a) Non-antibiotic treatment recommendations: Delivery formats and implications for parent resistance. *Social Science & medicine* 60 (5): 949–964. https://doi.org/10.1016/j.socscimed.2004.06.040

Stivers, Tanya (2005b) Parent resistance to physicians' treatment recommendations: One resource for initiating a negotiation of the treatment decision. *Health Communication* 18 (1): 41–74. https://doi.org/10.1207/s15327027hc1801_3

Suurmond, Jeanine and Conny Seeleman (2006) Shared decision-making in an intercultural context: Barriers in the interaction between physicians and immigrant patients. *Patient Education and Counseling* 60 (2): 253–259. https://doi.org/10.1016/j.pec.2005.01.012

Tebble, Helen (1999) The tenor of consultant physicians: Implications for medical interpreting. *The Translator* 5 (2): 179-200. https://doi.org/10.1080/13556509.1999.10799040

Wadensjö, Cecilia (1998) *Interpreting as Interaction*. Harlow, UK: Addison Wesley Longman.

Claudio Baraldi is Professor of Sociology of cultural and communicative processes at the University of Modena and Reggio Emilia, Italy. His research includes studies on intercultural communication, interlinguistic and intercultural mediation, conflict management and the development of techniques of dialogue. He has published several papers on dialogue interpreting in books and international journals, many with Laura Gavioli. With Laura Gavioli, he has also edited the volume *Coordinating Participation in Dialogue Interpreting* (John Benjamins, 2012). Address for correspondence: Dipartimento di Studi linguistici e culturali, Università di Modena e Reggio Emilia, Largo Sant'Eufemia 19, 41124 Modena, Italy. Email: claudio.baraldi@unimore.it

Laura Gavioli is Professor of English Language and Translation at the University of Modena and Reggio Emilia, Italy. Her work includes the study of spoken language in institutional settings, corpus studies for language learning and translation and the pragmatics of English–Italian interaction. She has been engaged in research exploring authentic data of interpreter-mediated conversations involving speakers of English and Italian, mainly in health-care settings. With Claudio Baraldi, she edited the volume *Coordinating Participation in Dialogue Interpreting* (John Benjamins, 2012). Address for correspondence: Dipartimento di Studi linguistici e culturali, Università di Modena e Reggio Emilia, Largo Sant'Eufemia 19, 41124 Modena, Italy.
Email: laura.gavioli@unimore.it

5 Involvement, trust and topic control in interpreter-mediated healthcare encounters

Cecilia Wadensjö

5.1 Introduction

Several articles published in the domain of medical encounters have concluded that the presence of an interpreter leads to less satisfactory communication. How come? One would presume that if a patient and a physician are unable or unwilling to communicate in a common language, they would appreciate the assistance of an interpreter. Nonetheless, research on patients' satisfaction with physician communication indicates that the presence of an interpreter tends to pull down patients' satisfaction rating. In order to problematize these results, Aranguri *et al.* (2006) suggest, as an alternative to having participants evaluate and rate communication, exploring patterns of communication that characterize interpreter-mediated encounters and the potential consequences of these patterns on the quality of the exchange between physicians and patients. Based on such an examination the authors found that 'the presence of an interpreter increases the difficulty of achieving good physician-patient communication' (Aranguri *et al.* 2006: 623). Moreover, they argue that this is the case regardless of the interpreter's level of training for their job and the physician's level of training for communication through interpreters, due to the complex nature of the interpreted situation. Still, they recommend that interpreters as well as physicians should get special training for this kind of situation in order 'to minimize conversational loss and maximize the information and relational exchange' (Aranguri *et al.* 2006: 623). After all, the presence of an interpreter is often the only available solution to an urgent communication problem. But what if physicians and patients do not perceive of one another as conversational partners? The present paper will address this elementary attitude issue and shed some light on its possible impact on the complexity of interpreter-mediated encounters.

Applying a dialogical view of language and mind (see e.g. Linell 2009 for a detailed outline of the theoretical framework of dialogism), the present study takes as a point of departure that interlocutors share responsibility for the messages communicated and for what is accomplished communicatively in social interaction. Moreover, as Heath and Luff (2012) convincingly argue, drawing on naturally occurring discourse data from medical encounters, participants' 'visible conduct often plays a crucial role both in the distribution and coordination of opportunities to participate, and in the structure of actions that participants are able and required to produce' (Heath and Luff 2012: 291 – for similar arguments specifically concerning interpreter-mediated encounters, see Krystallidou 2014.) This article explores *how*, precisely, participation is structured in two interpreter-mediated medical encounters. A detailed study of these encounters reveals that the primary participants' orientations *vis-à-vis* one another as conversational partners vary, in ways that have implications for the interpreter's performance and for the alignment between doctors and patients.

Section 2 provides a brief overview of research into interpreter-mediated medical encounters. In Section 3, the exchanges in sequences drawn from two authentic medical encounters are explored in detail, focusing on conditions for building rapport across language barriers. The concluding section discusses possible implications of monolingual participants not accepting each other as 'proper' conversational partners for the care provider's topic control, for the interpreter's involvement and for the establishment of mutual trust.

5.2 Studies of patient–doctor interaction

Much of the research on interaction in medical encounters concerns the ways in which medical practitioners control its content. Applying Mishler's (1984) distinction between the *voice of medicine* and the *voice of the lifeworld*, researchers have argued that doctors tend to ignore patients' mentioning of personal experiences, lay theories and concerns, and instead emphasize a strictly medical approach to physical and other problems. Doctors have been seen as eliciting information from patients that first and foremost complies with the needs of the care-providing body. In this way, it has been argued, the world of medicine as a modern technocratic system is cemented and maintained. Further, as Aronsson *et al.* (1995) demonstrate, the patient, being an active partner, tends to assist in maintaining the identified voice of medicine in medical encounters. The concept of patient-centred care was not as established in the early 1980s, when Mishler was writing, as it is today; however, his argument remains pertinent in that it will always take an effort by the doctor to maintain and balance the voice of medicine and the voice of the lifeworld. The medical expert's balancing of these 'voices' probably varies, due to cultural conventions as well as individual differences, but it is likely to always have an impact on the level of rapport he or she is able to establish with the patient. It lies beyond the scope of this article to explore this issue in detail, but the analyses below shed some light on various effects of practitioners' efforts to build rapport with patients whose language they do not speak.

Attitudes to interpreters in medical encounters

The literature on interpreted medical encounters has grown considerably in recent decades (for overviews, see Flores 2005; Pöchhacker 2006, 2016; Sleptsova *et al.* 2014), and a frequent topic is patient satisfaction, which is linked to issues of rapport, patient compliance and trust. Hadziabdic (2011), for instance, shows how the issue of trust was decisive for how medical staff, patients and relatives in her studies perceived those serving as interpreters and for how these groups evaluated the treatment in question.

A vast number of survey and interview studies have generated valuable insights into participants' attitudes and understandings of interpreting and interpreters. Asked to give their opinions about something they have experienced, informants also reveal their limited knowledge about what performing as an interpreter implies in terms of bilingual fluency, analytical skills and interpreting proficiencies. For instance, Hadziabdic and colleagues quote informants who argue against professional interpreting because, in their view, this consists of a 'literal and objective transfer of information', while they would prefer a more personal approach (Hadziabdic *et al.* 2014: 162).

The problem is that the reader is left with the impression that 'literal and objective transfer of information' is something that actually can and does take place, which is quite a misleading suggestion. For one thing, 'objective interpreting' is a contradiction in terms. Interpreting never happens without an interpreting subject – it is always an inherently subjective endeavour. Further, as the latest decades of studies on naturally occurring interpreter-mediated interaction show, interpreting spontaneous talk-in-interaction is hardly ever literal, because of discrepancies between different languages' formal structures and also because of the specific grammar of spoken interaction.

In survey and interview studies it is also often unclear what level of interpreter performance informants base their experiences upon – that is, whether they have encountered professionally trained interpreters, untrained language brokers or *ad hoc*, more or less bilingual medical staff. 'Interpreter' is a label used for all these categories. Also, individuals paid to carry out medical interpreting assignments (and who therefore are taken to be professionals) do not always have a relevant educational background. Formal interpreter training may not be available for them or, also when available, not required. Exploring and describing authentic regular medical encounters show that medical institutions in the US and in Germany respectively assign lay persons to perform interpreting (for the US e.g. Angelelli 2004, 2011; for Germany e.g. Meyer 2001, 2012 and Bührig and Meyer 2004).

Undoubtedly, it is much easier to communicate in one language (especially one's native tongue) than to consistently relay what others are saying, switching between two languages. This may partly explain why those performing as interpreters in the studies mentioned above frequently initiate side sequences in one language only. This is in particular done in order to negotiate with the patient the content of his or her contributions. As a result, the medical practitioner is kept waiting and prevented from gaining insight into which information, if any, originated in what the patient said and what the patient actually understood. In addition, this restricts the patient's and the doctor's possibility of aligning emotionally with one another, let alone explore one another's position on the subject matter.

Nevertheless, non-interpreted side sequences often seem to occur with the medical expert's tacit support. Physicians may expect interpreters to explain procedures for the patient (Angelelli 2004, 2011), or invite them to give advice on how to talk about potentially critical issues (Gavioli 2015) – treating the interpreter as their confidant (Hsieh 2006). Participants occasionally legitimize this approach with reference to doctors' and patients' different cultural backgrounds (Sleptsova *et al.* 2014). In a survey carried out among a large number of medical professionals, Felberg and Skaaden (2012) found that many informants ascribe problems encountered in interpreted conversations precisely to 'different cultures'. Yet, as the authors note,

> the use of the concept of 'culture' may lead to 'othering' of minority patients, may conceal rather than reveal communication problems, and may confuse the intersection between interpreters' and medical professionals' areas of expertise (Felberg and Skaaden 2012: 95).

The dynamics of interpreter-mediated medical encounters

Occasionally in healthcare studies, the interpreter is described as a tool that will be of practical use and efficient only if used correctly (e.g. Hsieh 2006, 2007; Pergert *et al.* 2008). This tool metaphor might seem attractive, as it draws attention to the responsibility of the person in charge. Yet, as Hsieh and Kramer argue, 'a utilitarian approach to the interpreter's role and functions may create interpersonal and ethical dilemmas that compromise the quality of care' (Hsieh and Kramer 2012: 158). Furthermore, it fails to capture the dynamics in interpreter-mediated medical encounters, where much complexity results from the involvement of three sense-making individuals whereof two do not speak a common language. Research on naturally occurring interpreting as interaction (Wadensjö 1992, 1998) has highlighted that interpreted conversations are co-constructed, tightly coordinated activities, in which participants' contributions are attributed meaning and purpose and that interpreters working in face-to-face encounters can be understood as having a dual task – that of rendering and coordinating others' talk, managing not only the content but simultaneously also, at some level, the progression of talk in interaction, or, to use Roy's (2000) terminology, managing the discourse flow. When assisted by an interpreter, monolingual medical staff – willingly or unwillingly, and irrespective of the interpreter's level of training – will have to delegate some responsibility for the content of the exchange and the progression of turn-taking (Sacks *et al.* 1974) to the bilingual person in the middle.

On involvement and topic control

The appropriate level of involvement is a frequent concern for professional interpreters. In a study of medical encounters where Spanish-speaking doctors met with non-Spanish-speaking patients, Valero-Garcés (2005) compares (1) monolingual encounters, where the patient speaks very limited English or Spanish, (2) bilingual encounters, mediated by an *ad hoc* bilingual person and (3) bilingual encounters, mediated by a person with some training as a hospital interpreter. As the author remarks, the Type 1 and Type 2 encounters share some features related to the use of certain communicative strategies, such as frequent questions, repetitions and reformulations, and these affect the general structure of the interview and the participants' involvement. The interpreter in the Type 3 encounters maintains an impartial role and uses specific strategies such as direct rendition of questions or asking for reformulation when they have difficulties, for example with terminology. Also, the trained interpreter uses the first person when talking on the primary participants' behalf, whereas the *ad hoc* interpreter tends to use the third person ('she says' etc.). As a consequence, the *ad hoc* interpreter's involvement as a participant is time and again put to the fore, while the primary participants are objectified, as it were, by being talked *about* rather than *to*.

These and other studies demonstrate the double-edged power of individuals assigned to perform as interpreters. On the one hand, they facilitate the monolingual parties' communication; but on the other, their performance can potentially also disempower both patients and care providers if restricting them from engaging in mutual communication, either by imposing personal ideas of what knowledge is necessary or unnecessary for them to share, or by failing to grasp something that was said, or by being unable to reproduce what was said in the other language. Yet even if the interpreter's position and competence are crucial, communication depends not on this one individual alone.

Davidson (1998, 2000) and Angelelli (2011), exploring data collected in Californian hospitals, noted that hospital-based Spanish–English interpreters were encouraged by physicians and administrators to keep the time spent in consultations to a minimum. This can partly explain, says Davidson, why interpreters in his study tend to assume the role of gatekeeper, editing or omitting patients' contributions to the encounter so as to 'keep the patient "on track" and keep the interview moving quickly' (Davidson 1998: v). As is shown in his data, this also implies favouring the voice of medicine (Mishler 1984).

5.3 Two medical encounters

The exchanges explored in this article are drawn from a large corpus of audio-recorded, interpreted encounters, interviews and field notes, collected in Swedish institutional – medical and legal – settings. The languages involved were Swedish, Spanish and Russian. The material was collected after ethics approval and with informed consent. The overall aim was to investigate the communicative peculiarities and particularities of interpreter-mediated encounters and to develop a theoretical framework for exploring interpreting as interaction (Wadensjö 1992). The two encounters explored here are similar in many ways, but differ substantially when it comes to the primary parties' ways of attending to one another as conversational partners, which is why they are selected for this study.

The study at hand involves two interpreters with a special Swedish authorization in medical interpreting (for further explanation, see Idh 2007). These interpreters also have similar levels of professional education: university diplomas in public service interpreting (three semesters of studies, including interpreting techniques and interpreting ethics) and more than five years of practice in medical, social security and legal encounters. Principally, they both act in the manner expected of interpreters in what Valero-Garcés (2005) calls Type 3 encounters, as described above. A core principle for such interpreters is that primary participants should have equal access to everything said in their presence.

The first two excerpts are drawn from an encounter where a Spanish-speaking woman living in Sweden is meeting a gynaecologist. Three days earlier, she gave birth to a baby and her delivery had been exceptionally difficult. On the day in question, she is to be discharged from the hospital, but prior to that she will have a final check-up.

'Any thoughts?'

Excerpt 1 starts eight minutes into the conversation. In total, the check-up took almost half an hour, much longer than the gynaecologist had anticipated, as she mentioned in the *post hoc* interview. The mother was concerned about her poor physical state after the delivery and also, it turned out, about the fact that she had not been given a caesarean section. The sequence begins right after the doctor's question in Swedish (*Any thoughts she wants to bring up before we end the conversation?*) followed by the interpreter's rendition in Spanish (*In general, do you have anything you'd like to ask about before we conclude the conversation?*). The non-idiomatic English translations provided below each turn reflect the pronounced spoken language, i.e., the fragmented character of the original talk. In print, this may seem rather confusing, but in oral communication, it may appear quite normal, not at all distracting. The transcripts include the conventional signs used in the field of interpreting studies to help analyse the interaction.

Excerpt 1: (Linköping Corpus G6: 5-6) D = Doctor; I = Interpreter; M = Mother

01 M: no, que:: en adelante igual se me
no, tha::t it'll probably be okay
02 pasa como está irritado y- a mí me
since it's irritated and the- my it's
03 arde la vagina me arde un poco.
burning the vagina burns a little.
04 una pequeña como que me pica aquí
it's slightly like its itching like here
05 arribita esa parte después me viene
up here this part and then there is
06 como una picazón yo pienso que-
like an itching I think that-
07 pienso que debe ser normal.
think that it should be normal.
08 I: ja de de- men därför de e också
well it it- but therefore it's also
det finns e:: antar jag att det är
there is eh, I guess that it's
09 lite irriterat, lite mycket irriterat
a bit irritated, a bit much irritated
10 eftersom det svider lite och se'n lite
because it stings a bit and then a bit
11 i närheten av vagina, det måste vara
close to the vagina, that must be
12 på grund av såna saker,
because of those kinds of things,
13 och så det finns e:n lite liten klåda,
and so there is a little small itching.
14 D: [mhm]
15 I: [lite] högre upp me:n
[*a bit*] *higher up bu:t*
16 D: [mhm]
17 I: [jag] antar att de e normalt.
[*I*] *assume that it's normal.*
18 M: o sea mi hija la tuve con cesárea

that is my girl I got her through
19 entonces es la primera vez que
caesarean this is the first time that
20 tengo un parto normal así
I have a normal childbirth like this
21 que por eso. no sé.
so that's why. don't know.
22 I: det andra barnet som jag hade det
the other child that I had it
23 var med kejsarsnitt, så
was through a caesarean section, so
24 det är första gången som jag har en
it's the first time that I have a
25 normal förlossning.
a normal delivery.
26 D: mm
27 I: så jag vet inte.
so I don't know.
28 D: näe, vi ska passa på å
well, we'll take the opportunity to
29 undersöka [så
examine [so

At the start of the excerpt, the doctor had signaled readiness to move on to the physical examination. Her question ahead of the extract, *Any thoughts she wants to bring up before we end the conversation?*, can be recognized as a means of initiating termination, not just of the current topic but also as a way of closing the conversation (Schegloff and Sacks 1973). Notably, while the doctor addresses the interpreter, saying *she wants*, the interpreter addresses the mother: *do you have*. Having heard the rendition, the mother starts speaking in the same weak voice as during the prior eight minutes. After an initial *no* she eventually expresses some thoughts. First, she comes up with certain doubts (*it'll probably be okay*, line 01), before going on to tentatively express concerns about her current condition (lines 02–07). The interpreter renders the mother's somewhat disjointed talk, not in all details, but reflecting some of its bitty character (lines 08–13, 15 and 17). The mother's talk is quite emotional, weak and distressed. The interpreter, however, speaking for her, talks in a much clearer and more distinct voice.

Elsewhere, I have suggested differentiating between the strategies of *relaying by displaying* (representing), and *relaying by replaying* (re-presenting), as a way of distinguishing between interpreters' various approaches to rendering the words of others (Wadensjö 1998: 239–248). If we see these approaches as two endpoints of a continuum, the interpreter's way of relaying in the above sequence has more of a relaying-by-displaying character, as she seeks to represent the mother's words without mirroring her emotionally coloured performative style. This implies that if the doctor focuses only on what the interpreter says, she might miss what the mother communicates with the tone and quality of her voice. Furthermore, if the doctor focuses on the interpreter as a conversational partner, she might miss what the mother communicates by her mere appearance. She is sitting on the edge of her chair, and her facial expression communicates distress when she occasionally and carefully changes her seating position.

Yet, looking further into the transcript, the doctor's rather softly spoken feedback *mhm* (lines 14 and 16), coming partly in parallel with the interpreter's talk (lines 15 and 17), may be a sign of her paying attention to the mother's expression of disappointment. It may be unclear to her, however, whether or not the mother pays mutual attention. The mother goes on talking in her grumbling voice, now comparing her recent and previous experiences of childbirth (lines 18–21). This was her second child and her first natural delivery: the first child was born in Chile, where she had had a caesarean section. The doctor again confirms attentiveness (line 26) to the interpreter's renditions of this statement (lines 22–25) and then makes a new effort to bring the conversation to an end, mentioning the physical examination that she had planned for the mother today (lines 28–29).

Notably, the doctor did not seem to accept the mother as her proper interlocutor, and nor did the mother seem to accept the doctor in such a role either. The mother has something to say regarding the doctor's *any thoughts?* question. She shares thoughts about her present and previous experiences of childbirth, albeit by consistently turning to the interpreter. The interpreter, in turn, confirms with quick glances that she is listening and understanding, while relaying the mother's talk into Swedish. Most of the time, however, the interpreter looks straight ahead or moves her gaze towards the doctor, seeking to redirect, as it were, the mother's gaze from herself to the doctor. In other words, she uses both verbal and non-verbal means to promote a more direct contact between the other two.

'Don't want any more children?'

Excerpt 2 begins where Excerpt 1 ends, with the mother's expression of uncertainty upon the gynaecologist's suggestion to move on to the physical examination. In this sequence, lines 35–41 are particularly interesting from the point of view of topic shift and participant involvement. As became apparent in the *post hoc* interview, the doctor had not at all foreseen the topic of caesarean section, which was introduced by the mother. It started in the sequence shown in Excerpt 1, was firmly established right after the sequence shown in Excerpt 2 and was eventually discussed at length.

Excerpt 2: (Linköping Corpus G6:6)

31 M: despacito si e:::h porque
gentle okay e:::h because

32 I: mm, mycket försiktigt.
mm, very carefully.

33 D: [jaa, jag vet
[yeah, I know

34 M: [(xxxx)

35 I: si ya lo sé (.) jag är så nervös.
yes I know this (.) I'm so nervous.

36 M: todo lo que me ha pasado ya de
everything that's already happened to

37 mamá así que::: ((light laughter))
me as a mother so::: ((light laughter))

38 I: med allt som jag har gått igenom så::
with everything I've gone through so::

39 jag vill inte ha mer.
I don't want to have more.

40 D: vill inte ha flera barn? eller.
don't want any more children? or.

41 I: no quieres tener más hijos tampoco?
don't you want any more children either?

42 M: no ahora. al menos que:::
not now. unless:::

43 I: inte:: nu.
no::t now.

The mother says *gently okay e:::h because* (line 31), which is rendered as *mm, very carefully.* (line 32) – that is, as a somewhat disambiguated version of her statement. The doctor confirms that she knows (line 33), while the mother, talking in overlap, has more to say. Notably, the interpreter renders their talk in order of appearance, demonstrating the division of voices by means of a distinct pause between two chunks of talk (line 35). The mother goes on to produce some more talk (*everything that's already happened to me as a mother so:::*), followed by a light nervous laughter (lines 36–37). The interpreter most likely reads this as a request for saving her from more pain, relaying it as *with everything I've gone through so:: I don't want to have more* (lines 38–39) – that is, in a semantically more complete form than the mother's original expression, yet with a similar level of vagueness.

At this point, the doctor asks, *don't want any more children? or?* (line 40), showing that she is sensitive to the mother's signs of distress. In an interpreter-mediated encounter, a question designed to check what was just said – a so-called repair initiation (Schegloff 2007: 102) – potentially addresses both the interpreter and the person the interpreter has just spoken for. In principle, the interpreter at this point could have relayed this as a repair initiation that would have allowed, or urged, the mother to specify what she had just meant to say. But the interpreter renders the gynaecologist's *don't want any more children? or?* (line 40) as *don't you want any more children either?* (line 41).

Listening to the recording, it seems unlikely that the interpreter could have misheard what the doctor said. Looking at the entire encounter, the quoted rendition (line 41) seems rather to follow a certain general tendency. In the interpreter's version, the doctor's question is phrased as a question from someone who is understanding and attending closely to the mother's complaints and who is ready to hear more about these, rather than someone who is asking about the meaning of certain words. Again, the interpreter seems to be oriented towards prompting the primary participants' attention to one another as conversational partners.

Face-work and vagueness

The first two examples in this article may illustrate how *face-work* (Goffman 1967) can have a considerable impact on the organization and thereby also on the content of an interpreter-mediated conversation. 'Face-work' means measures taken to counteract possible risks of hurting others' feelings by behaviour that might be taken as disrespectful and that might risk loss in self-respect (Goffman 1967:12). Vagueness is a typical strategy for saving face. This can partly explain why the mother did not address the practitioner directly, but rather might have expected the interpreter to filter, as it were, her concern and critique.

To the interpreter, vagueness is in itself an additional challenge. For one thing, it is quite demanding just to follow and to memorize vaguely formulated utterances. Second, it can be socially demanding to repeat a vaguely formulated utterance in a vague way, not only because the interpreter risks being understood as the source of this vagueness, but also because the voicing of someone else's vagueness can be understood as parodying them, in other words as being quite face-threatening. Due to emotional content, the interpreter sometimes goes for *displaying* rather than *replaying* the speaker's performative style. The selected approach, it seems, depends on the current context, the institutional setting, the constellation of people and, not least, the primary participants' readiness to attend to each other as conversational partners.

The third and last example below will demonstrate, by way of contrast, how vagueness and fragmented speech do not necessarily jeopardize efficient communication between the primary participants. Excerpt 3 is drawn from an encounter where another young, dissatisfied mother meets an educational nurse at a Swedish childcare clinic. Semantically, the exchange was not less complex than Excerpts 1–2 for the interpreter to memorize and convey in the other language. Socially, however, the situation was quite different, in that the primary participants' orientation towards one another as conversational partners was evident from the start. Moreover, they largely seem to have shared expectations and viewpoints concerning the purpose of their meeting and the interpreter's mandate in it.

'This worries me a lot'

The encounter took place in a small neighbourhood clinic, to where a young Russian-speaking mother had brought her baby girl to ask for advice. The analysed sequence mostly consists of the mother's talk and the interpreter's renditions. The care provider's involvement is seen only in frequent feedback tokens, indicating her active listening. The extract (Excerpt 3) begins when the mother has just brought up the problem of 'the infection' which she sees on her daughter's leg. The mother appears to be unsettled by the information she has received so far, wondering what it is that has irritated her baby more or less from birth.

Excerpt 3: (Linköping Corpus G42:13-14)

01 M: да то есть буквально- и мы- в
yes that is literally- and we- (.) at
02 начале у нее- приходила-

the beginning she had- I came-
03 мне это очень беспокоит.
I'm very worried about this.
04 I: mm
05 M: [я все время приходила к врачу.
[I've all the time come to the doctor
06 что это? они говорят, все хорошо,
what's this? they say, everything's okay,
07 все хорошо (.) а я же видела.
everything's okay but I saw, didn't I
08 [что-то такое
[something so
09 I: [mhm,] mm å ja har varit,
[mhm] mm and I've been,
10 väldigt orolig hela tiden, jag har,
very worried all the time, I've,
11 frågat läkaren eller
asked the doctor or
12 N: [aa
[yeah
13 I: [e::h] sjuksköterskorna hela
e::h the nurses all the
14 tiden. va- va kan de bero [på?
time. wha- what may be the [reason.
15 N: [aa
[yeah
16 I: a de e okej,
well that's okay,
17 [de e okej.
[that's okay.
18 N: [mhm
19 I: de e inget å oroa sig [för.
this is nothing to worry [about.
20 N: [mhm, aa-
21 M: то есть- а это,
that is- but this,
N: [de va,
[that was,
23 M: [вообще бывает? вот что это такое.
[in general this happens? so what is
24 [потому что я:::
[this. because I:::
25 N: [problemet-
[the problem-
26 I: [men eh: det händer alltså? å
[but er: it happens that is? and

27 va e det egentligen?
what is it actually?
28 [vad kan] det bero på?
[what is] the reason?
29 N: [ja de-]
[yes it-]

In this excerpt, the mother tells about previous experiences from conversations with healthcare personnel. Her account takes the form of a staged dialogue between herself and those she had met. She paints a picture of past encounters with healthcare staff members, where she *all the time* (line 05) has been asking *what's this?* (line 06), while they have answered *everything's okay, everything's okay* (lines 06–07). Obviously, the protagonists quoted from the past potentially also include the immediate past; that is, the present encounter. The mother is clearly dissatisfied with the nurse's explanation concerning the baby's leg.

The interpreter in turn relays the mother's staging of characters, using semantic means similar to those utilized by the original speaker. She gives voice to an *I*, signifying the mother in interaction at past occasions with members of the medical staff. She first quotes the mother's lines, until *wha- what may be the reason?*, lines 09–14) and then those of the caring staff/the nurse (*well that's okay, that's okay.*, lines 16–17). Notably, the interpreter specifies the meaning of *well that's okay, that's okay*, saying *this is nothing to worry about* (line 19), which answers directly to how the mother introduces her story (*I'm very worried about this*, line 03). The mother's narration ends in a question which in view of the described past dialogues could be read as quite a critical comment. She has still not received a satisfactory answer to her question about her daughter's leg. The interpreter relays this, and the nurse subsequently explains that what is seen on the baby's leg is not an infection but an abscess, the body's own protection mechanism, which is quite normal and which will soon disappear. The issue, which relates to medicine as well as the lifeworld, is intensively discussed, subsequently settled after some more rounds of talk and then dropped.

Communication and mutual trust

The exchange cited in Excerpt 3 took 28 seconds. It contains a mini-story conveying worry, accumulated over numerous encounters with medical institutions. Worry as a dominating emotional expression colours the interpreter's contributions as well. She also speaks at about the same speed as the mother, communicating, like the prior speaker, frustration and worry, also with the tone of her voice. The interpreter largely employs the strategy of relaying by replaying, counting on the primary participants' orientation towards one another as their respective proper interlocutor and relying on her ability to make it clear that she is conveying the mother's and not her own uncertainty, using modulation of voice, emphasis and gaze direction as communicative resources to mark the distinction between the speaking self (the interpreter) and the meaning other (the mother). No doubt, the interpreter's need to mark this distinction depends on the primary participants' orientation to one another and to the interpreter.

The relative closeness between the mother's and the interpreter's talk is clearly supported by the nurse's bodily displayed involvement. The 'tightness' of discourse has a correspondence in the physical space created between the participants. When the mother sits down in the middle of the small office, the nurse immediately brings her own chair from behind her desk and places herself very close to her. The object of conversation – the baby – is present for her to see and reach. The mother, in turn, displays anxiousness to share her worries with the nurse.

The primary participants often talk in overlap, and parallel talk with the interpreter's utterances is frequent. The parallel talk does not seem to obstruct interaction, but rather the opposite. Turns are exchanged with high frequency. Eventually, the exchanges turn out to involve a lot of smiles and laughter. The tense atmosphere (in Excerpt 3) was quite temporary. The meeting, planned for 20 minutes, also took this time. Arguably, the primary participants' trust in the interpreter's ability to mediate accurately, and not least their trust in their orientation to each other as their 'proper' conversational partner, facilitated the professional interpreter's job and eventually the establishment of common focus, shared involvement and efficient communication.

5.4 Concluding discussion

In several brochures and guidebooks on how to work with interpreters, I have read that medical staff must realize that 'word-for-word translation will not be sufficient' (Bischoff and Loutan 2008: 25). Even a cursory look at the spontaneous spoken interaction transcribed above makes it evident that relaying word-for-word simply would not make sense. The everyday notion of professional interpreting as word-for-word translation does not correspond to reality. Yet beginners in the profession typically render fractions of talk word-for-word, as they tend to stick too closely to the source-language structure.

The proficient interpreter is trained to focus relatively more on content than on form, not only because different languages tend to organize reality into somewhat different semantic fields, but also because delivery is expected without delay as the conversation unfolds. This puts considerable pressure on the interpreter's ability to focus, analyse and produce instant renditions of what was just said. Interpreting inherently implies taking content that was presented in one language and redesigning it in another language for a particular recipient or recipients, in a specific context. The task demands empathy, personal integrity and knowledge of the subject matter and of the logics of the institution, as well as linguistic and interpreting skills.

Professional interpreters are expected to be not only fluent in their working languages but also seamless in their practice of switching between these languages. They are expected to be able to render any utterance, whether composed of fragmented gibberish or eloquent rhetoric, and, on top of that, to be able to manage the common discourse flow without disturbing the primary participants in their speech production. In practice, of course, peoples' verbal performance varies. This goes for interpreters as well as for patients and doctors. Meeting someone whose language you do not understand, you do not always know how to express your thoughts when asked to do so. Patients as well as practitioners may be counting on the interpreter not just to render their talk, but also to guide them in what to say. (This is why interpreters are trained to briefly present their specific mandate and responsibility at the onset of an encounter.)

The two encounters discussed in this article involve both similar and various difficulties for the interpreters. In both, a young migrant mother was visiting respectively a Swedish maternity ward and a childcare ward. Both mothers were critical of previously offered treatment. So as not to be face-threatening, their criticism was expressed quite vaguely, which inevitably led to challenges for the interpreter. For interpreters, it may require extra discipline to refrain from clarifying something ambiguously expressed (Wadensjö 1998: 159; Lee 2009). Due to cognitive constraints, it is inherently difficult to recapitulate exactly and repeat fragmented speech in any language. Also, due to social constraints, interpreters may hesitate to even make an effort to render a speaker's disjointed or vague talk in the same vague style, since they risk being understood as either the source of the incoherence or as parodying the speaker. Interpreters who experience that mutual trust is at stake tend to refrain from even trying to relay fragmented talk as fragmented in order not to further jeopardize the participants' trust in each other as interlocutors and in themselves as accurate interpreters.

Involvement is interactively accomplished

Arguably, mutual trust was indeed at issue more or less from the start in the encounter represented in Excerpts 1 and 2. The mother consistently tended to address the interpreter rather than the gynaecologist, who also addressed the interpreter and spoke to the mother only indirectly. The primary participants' stances were evident not only from what they said, but also from the way they positioned themselves physically in relation to one another and the interpreter.

The rendition discussed in relation to Excerpt 2 (line 32) illustrates how the interpreter often tried to promote mutual focus between the two primary parties. Tacitly promoting them to accept one another as each other's 'proper' conversational partner, the interpreter also avoids putting focus on herself as a (mis)understanding subject. Positioning herself as someone 'just interpreting' the mother's and the doctor's words, the interpreter worked on establishing the parties' sense of 'being with' one another, even though the exchange, at a certain level, was carried out as two parallel conversations, one between the interpreter and the doctor and the other between the interpreter and the mother.

Eventually, however, their conversation developed around what seemed to be the mother's main concern – her disappointment at not having been offered a caesarean section. The practitioner found a way to meet this, in a way that proved satisfactory to both. The mother left the hospital knowing more about the pros and cons of caesarean sections; but the encounter took much longer than anticipated and the practitioner's visible conduct probably did not convey to the mother that she did indeed care about the mother's worries, and that she was indeed prepared to balance the voice of medicine and the voice of the lifeworld.

In the encounter in Excerpt 3, conversely, the Russian-speaking interpreter, although she had to deal with vague and emotional talk, was much closer to relaying by replaying than the Spanish-speaking interpreter in Excerpts 1 and 2. Obviously, this is partly explained by her proficiency in terms of bilingual vocabulary, translation fluency, speed and sense of timing, but the efficiency of communication in the constellation of people represented in Excerpt 3 is clearly also due to the parties' acceptance of one another as proper conversational parties. In order to build trust with patients whose language they do not share, care providers may need to be aware of, engage with and rely on, not only interpreters, but also on their own various resources for communication across languages.

Transcription conventions

:::	Prolongation of the sound preceding (more colons = loner prolongation).
-	Cut-off or self-interruption.
[	Point of overlap onset.
(.)	Dot in brackets indicates 'micropause', audible but not readily measurable. ordinarily less than 0.2 of a second.
(xxx)	The letter 'x' in parentheses indicates inaudible speech.
.	A falling, or final intonation contour.
,	'Continuing' intonation, not necessarily a clause boundary.
?	Rising intonation, not necessarily a question.
<u>all</u>	Underline indicates stress.

References

Angelelli, Claudia V. (2004) *Medical Interpreting and Cross-Cultural Communication*. Cambridge: Cambridge University Press. https://doi.org/10.1017/CBO9780511486616

Angelelli, Claudia V. (2011) 'Can you ask her about chronical illnesses, diabetes and all that?' In C. Alvstad, A. Hild and E. Tiselius (eds) *Methods and Strategies of Process Research*, 231–246. Amsterdam: John Benjamins. https://doi.org/10.1075/btl.94.17ang

Aranguri, Cesar, Brad Davidson and Robert Ramirez (2006) Patterns of communication through interpreters: A detailed sociolinguistic analysis. *Journal of General Internal Medicine* 21 (6): 623–629. https://doi.org/10.1111/j.1525-1497.2006.00451.x

Aronsson, Karin, Ullabeth Sätterlund Larsson and Roger Säljö (1995) Clinical diagnosis and the joint construction of a medical voice. In Ivana Marková and Robert M. Farr (eds) *Representations of Health, Illness and Handicap*, 131–144. Chur, Switzerland: Harwood Academic Publishers.

Bischoff, Alexander and Louis Loutan (2008) *Other Words, Other Meanings: A Guide to Health Care Interpreting in International Settings*. Translated by M. Gubitz and C. White. Geneva: Hôpitaux Universitaires de Genève.

Bührig, Kristin and Bernd Meyer (2004) *Ad hoc*-interpreting and the achievement of communicative purposes in doctor-patient communication. In Juliane House and Jochen Rehbein (eds) *Multilingual Communication*, 43–62. Amsterdam: John Benjamins.

Davidson, Brad (1998) *Interpreting Medical Discourse: A Study of Cross-Linguistic Communication in the Hospital Clinic*. Unpublished doctoral dissertation, Stanford University, Stanford, CA.

Davidson, Brad (2000) The interpreter as institutional gatekeeper: The social-linguistic role of interpreters in Spanish-English medical discourse. *Journal of Sociolinguistics* 4 (3): 379–405. https://doi.org/10.1111/1467-9481.00121

Felberg, Tatjana R. and Hanne Skaaden (2012) The (de)construction of culture in interpreter-mediated medical discourse. *Linguistica Antverpiensia* (New Series) 11: 95–112.

Flores, Glenn (2005) The impact of medical interpreter services on the quality of health care: A systematic review. *Medical Care Research and Review* 62 (3): 255–299. https://doi.org/10.1177/1077558705275416

Gavioli, Laura (2015) On the distribution of responsibility in treating critical issues in interpreter-mediated medical consultations: The case of 'le spieghi(amo)'. *Journal of Pragmatics* 76: 169–180. https://doi.org/10.1016/j.pragma.2014.12.001

Goffman, Erving (1967) *Interactional Ritual: Essays on Face-to-Face Behaviour.* New York: Pantheon Books.

Hadziabdic, Emina (2011) *The Use of Interpreter[s] in Healthcare: Perspectives of Individuals, Healthcare Staff and Families*. Unpublished doctoral dissertation, Linnaeus University, Växjö, Sweden.

Hadziabdic, Emina, Björn Albin, Kristiina Heikkilä and Katarina Hjelm (2014) Family members' experiences of the use of interpreters in healthcare. *Primary Health Care Research & Development* 15 (2): 156–169. https://doi.org/10.1017/S1463423612000680

Heath, Christian and Paul Luff (2012) Embodied action and organizational activity. In Jack Sidnell and Tanya Stivers (eds) *The Handbook of Conversation Analysis*, 283–307. Chichester, UK: Wiley-Blackwell. https://doi.org/10.1002/9781118325001.ch14

Hsieh, Elaine (2006) Conflicts in how interpreters manage their roles in provider–patient interactions. *Social Science & Medicine* 62 (3): 721–730. https://doi.org/10.1016/j.socscimed.2005.06.029

Hsieh, Elaine (2007) Interpreters as co-diagnosticians: Overlapping roles and services between providers and interpreters. *Social Science & Medicine* 64 (4): 924–937. https://doi.org/10.1016/j.socscimed.2006.10.015

Hsieh, Elaine and Eric M. Kramer (2012) Medical Interpreters as tools: Dangers and challenges in the utilitarian approach to interpreters' role and functions. *Patient Education and Counseling* 89 (1): 158–162. https://doi.org/10.1016/j.pec.2012.07.001

Idh, Leena (2007) The Swedish system of authorizing interpreters. In Cecilia Wadensjö, Birgitta Englund Dimitrova and Anna-Lena Nilsson (eds) *The Critical Link 4: Professionalisation of Interpreting in the Community*, 135–138. Amsterdam: John Benjamins. https://doi.org/10.1075/btl.70.16idh

Krystallidou, Demi (2014) Gaze and body orientation as an apparatus for patient inclusion into/exclusion from a patient-centred framework of communication. *Interpreter and Translator Trainer* 8 (3): 399–417. https://doi.org/10.1080/1750399X.2014.972033

Lee, Jieun (2009) Interpreting inexplicit language during courtroom examination. *Applied Linguistics* 30 (1): 93–114. https://doi.org/10.1093/applin/amn050

Linell, Per (2009) *Rethinking Language, Mind and World Dialogically: Interactional and Contextual Theories of Human Sense-Making.* Charlotte, NC: Information Age Publishing.

Meyer, Bernd (2001) How untrained interpreters handle medical terms. In Ian Mason (ed.) *Triadic Exchanges: Studies in Dialogue Interpreting*, 87–106. Manchester: St. Jerome.

Meyer, Bernd (2012) *Ad hoc* interpreting for partially language-proficient patients: Participation in multilingual constellations. In Claudio Baraldi and Laura Gavioli (eds) *Coordinating Participation in Dialogue Interpreting*, 99–113. Amsterdam: John Benjamins. https://doi.org/10.1075/btl.102.05mey

Mishler, Elliot G. (1984) *The Discourse of Medicine: Dialectics in Medical Interviews.* Norwood, NJ: Ablex.

Pergert, Pernilla, Solvig Ekblad, Karin Enskär and Olle Björk (2008) Bridging obstacles to transcultural caring relationships: Tools discovered through interviews with staff in pediatric oncology care. *European Journal of Oncology Nursing* 12: 35–43. https://doi.org/10.1016/j.ejon.2007.07.006

Pöchhacker, Franz (2006) Research and methodology in healthcare interpreting. *Linguistica Antverpiensia* (New Series) 5: 135–160.

Pöchhacker, Franz (2016) *Introducing Interpreting Studies* (2nd revised edition) London: Routledge. https://doi.org/10.4324/9781315649573

Roy, Cynthia B. (2000) *Interpreting as a Discourse Process.* New York: Oxford University Press.

Sacks, Harvey, Emanuel A. Schegloff and Gail Jefferson (1974) A simplest systematics for the organization of turn-taking for conversation. *Language* 50 (4, Part 1): 696–735. https://doi.org/10.1353/lan.1974.0010

Schegloff, Emanuel A. (2007) *Sequence Organization in Interaction.* Cambridge: Cambridge University Press. https://doi.org/10.1017/CBO9780511791208

Schegloff, Emanuel A. and Harvey Sacks (1973) Opening up closings. *Semiotica* 8 (4): 289–327. https://doi.org/10.1515/semi.1973.8.4.289

Sleptsova, Marina, Gertrud Hofer, Naser Morina and Wolf Langewitz (2014) The role of the health care interpreter in a clinical setting: A narrative review. *Journal of Community Health Nursing* 31: 167–184. https://doi.org/10.1080/07370016.2014.926682

Valero-Garcés, Carmen (2005) Doctor-patient communication in dyadic and triadic exchanges. *Interpreting* 7 (2): 193–210. https://doi.org/10.1075/intp.7.2.04val

Wadensjö, Cecilia (1992) *Interpreting as Interaction: On Dialogue-Interpreting in Immigration Hearings and Medical Encounters.* Doctoral dissertation, Linköping University, Linköping.

Wadensjö, Cecilia (1998) *Interpreting as Interaction.* Harlow, UK: Addison Wesley Longman.

Cecilia Wadensjö is Professor of Interpreting and Translation Studies at Stockholm University, Sweden. She has published extensively on interpreter-mediated social interaction, drawing on recordings of naturally occurring discourse data and exploring interpreting in medical, legal, broadcasted and other institutional encounters. Her publications include the widely cited monograph *Interpreting as Interaction* (1998, Addison Wesley Longman; reprinted 2014, Routledge). Address for correspondence: Institute for Interpreting and Translation Studies, Department of Swedish Language and Multilingualism, Stockholm University, SE-106 91 Stockholm, Sweden. Email: cecilia.wadensjo@su.se

6 Mutual (mis)understanding in interpreting in consultations between Turkish immigrant patients and Dutch general practitioners

Sione Twilt, Ludwien Meeuwesen,
Jan D. ten Thije & Hans Harmsen

Dedication

We dedicate this article to the memory of our colleague, Ludwien Meeuwesen.

6.1 Introduction

The present study focuses on the communicative actions of informal interpreters in interaction with Dutch general practitioners (GPs) and Turkish immigrant patients. The general aim is to gain insight into the quality of informal interpreting in the medical trialogue. The Netherlands has a multi-ethnic population: 22% is foreign-born, of which 56% is non-Western, with origins in places such as Suriname, Turkey and Morocco (Centraal Bureau voor de Statistiek [CBS] 2015). Most of these immigrants live in large cities, which is reflected in urban GPs' practices.

The multicultural contacts in medical encounters are often complicated by language barriers (Flores 2005; Meeuwesen *et al.* 2006) and also by differing cultural views and perceptions about illness and health (Kleinman 1980). Consequently, good mutual understanding and rapport between doctor and patient is more difficult to realize in intercultural medical settings (Harmsen 2003). Mutual understanding here refers to the patient's and the physician's awareness of each other's perspectives (Kleinman 1980) – for good-quality care, such mutual understanding is a prerequisite, as patients need to understand their physicians and they themselves need to be understood. Harmsen (2003) showed that poor mutual understanding between GPs and patients in the Rotterdam area was much higher among immigrant patients than Dutch patients (33% versus 13%). Besides patients' age and education, it was mainly their poor Dutch language proficiency which contributed to this low level of mutual understanding. In the Harmsen study, over 50% of immigrant patients had poor language proficiency in Dutch.

GPs have a central role in health care in the Netherlands, and their role includes a gatekeeping function: each doctor takes care of approximately 2500 patients, and specialists are only visited after referral by a GP. There are local foundations who finance formal interpreters for GPs. In daily practice, though, the majority of immigrants bring informal interpreters to the GPs' practices. It is estimated that patients bring interpreters to 20% of all Dutch GP consultations, at least in the large cities.

The present study is about the process of informal interpreting, focusing on the communicative actions of informal interpreters in interaction with GPs and patients. The aim is to gain insight into the advantages and disadvantages of using informal interpreters: which role-taking will an informal interpreter perform?; what kinds of miscommunication occur?; and under which conditions will the communication be successful? First, we contextualize the study by discussing the differences between formal and informal interpreters, the preferred roles and identities of interpreters, and then the causes of miscommunication.

Formal and informal interpreters

When patients and doctors do not share a common language, the use of interpreters is essential to realize effective communication. An often-made distinction is between formal and informal interpreters (e.g. Knapp-Potthoff and Knapp 1986, 1987; Bührig *et al.* 2009; Evrin and Meyer 2016; see also Zendedel 2017). Formal interpreters are trained professionals who are recruited through the institution, while informal interpreters tend to be family members, partners or friends who join the patients. Although a predominantly negative attitude exists regarding the use of informal interpreters, linguistic literature demonstrates that there is actually little difference in tasks and discourse structures between both types of interpreters (Bührig and Rehbein 1996; Apfelbaum 1998; ten Thije 2009). Differences refer mainly to non-linguistic characteristics such as the status, payment and education of the interpreter (Apfelbaum 1998). However, formal interpreters are trained in (medical) interpreting and are therefore more familiar with institutional constraints and purposes, as well as with specific institutional knowledge, including vocabulary. Doctors are therefore more inclined towards preferring this type of interpreting (Robb and Greenhalgh 2005). Patients, on the other hand, seem to prefer using a family member while talking to their doctor, because they feel they are better and can be advocates for their requests (Green *et al.* 2005).

Interpreter roles and identities

Interpreters may differ from each other in the ways they interpret and the roles they take (Wadensjö 1998; Bolden 2000; Bot 2005). An interpreter reproduces the communicative actions of the primary speakers, and by doing so not only provides a translation but also changes or characterizes the formulations (Bührig and Rehbein 1996). The translation may not be literal: the interpreter may dilate the communicative actions of the primary speakers, which is partly due to the large amount of internal, or mental, activities interpreters have to undertake. Formal interpreters seem to have developed these activities more than informal interpreters; they are more experienced in understanding the primary speakers and at the same time reproducing their words for the hearer.

Adopting a conversation analytical approach, Bot (2005) argues that interpreters seem to have difficulties in translating the language of the primary speakers precisely. She identifies two approaches to interpreting, that represent two poles of a continuum: the *translation-machine* model, in which the interpreter is present as a non-person who gives equivalent translations, and the *liberal interactive* model, in which the interpreter takes an interactive stance towards the interpreter-mediated medical encounter, leading to an accumulation of tasks (e.g. providing equivalent translations, contributing to the structure of the medical encounter, functioning as a cultural broker, etc.). It appears that interpreters cannot always act like a translation-machine model; in fact, they tend to participate as a third interlocutor during the interaction.

Wadensjö (1998) also states that the interpreter does not function as a translation machine, but rather participates in the interaction process on his or her own account. She discerns three roles that the interpreter can take on within the interaction: reporter, recapitulator and responder. The interpreter as *reporter* aims to translate the utterance of the primary speaker literally, which resembles the translation-machine model. The *recapitulator* changes the original utterance but aims for the content remains the same; such changes may contribute to increasing understanding between the primary speakers since the interpreter anticipates potential misunderstandings between the primary speakers. The *responder* role can be found when the interpreter reacts directly to an utterance of the primary speaker as an interlocutor without any translation taking place at all. These roles contribute to achieving mutual understanding in different ways. If we consider the responder role, one of the primary speakers is excluded from the communication. Because no translation is being rendered, a dyadic communication takes place, also called 'side-talk activity' (Wadensjö 1998). Private chats occur in the triadic interaction, which can have an effect on the communication between the three participants. In situations like medical encounters, the side-talk activity between the patient and the informal interpreter often causes the doctor to experience a feeling of exclusion (Rosenberg *et al.* 2007).

In health care, physicians generally do recognize these interpreter roles. They expect interpreters to be not only translators, but also to serve as cultural brokers and intercultural mediators in the case of formal interpreters or as caregivers in the case of informal interpreters (Knapp-Potthoff and Knapp 1986, 1987; Rosenberg *et al.* 2007; ten Thije 2009; see also Baraldi and Gavioli 2016). Informal interpreters also have useful additional information about the patient and his/her symptoms. From physicians' perspective, informal interpreters can be helpful in establishing good contact with the whole family. The disadvantage of informal interpreters might be that they may also have their own agenda in being present as a third party (Rosenberg *et al.* 2008).

Hasselkus (1992) distinguishes three roles for informal interpreters, drawing on the context of geriatrics and their caregivers: *facilitator*, in which the family member addresses the linguistic aspects of the patient's communication and increases understanding between doctor and patient; *intermediary*, where the family member functions as a cultural broker by focusing on linguistic and cultural understanding; and *direct source*, in which the family member is mostly a substitute for the patient. These roles are shown in more detail in Table 6.1.

Table 6.1 Characteristics of third-party interpreter roles: facilitator, intermediary and direct source (derived from Hasselkus 1992).

Facilitator	Intermediary	Direct source
Prompting, clarifying, correcting to increase patient's communication skills.	Answering doctor's direct questions about the patient.	Answering doctor's direct questions about patient
Explaining, repeating, paraphrasing to increase patient's and doctor's understanding.	Questioning doctor on behalf of the patient.	Questioning doctor about patient on his own account
	Questioning patient for doctor.	Volunteering, adding facts and information
	Volunteering, adding facts and information.	
	Checking with patient or doctor on facts and information	

In sum, all interpreters whether formal or informal seem to have an influence on medical encounters, although there is great variation. They at times translate precisely what the primary speakers say, but at other times may delete, expand or change utterances. Moreover, they can temporarily exclude a primary speaker from the interaction. The categories of interpreter roles suggested by Wadensjö (1998) and Hasselkus (1992) are largely comparable and recognized by physicians.

Miscommunication and causes

Roberts *et al.* (2005) describe in detail the communication problems in immigrant patient–doctor interaction in London GP surgeries. Different cultural backgrounds may mean differing ways of structuring information and of managing the encounter, due to sociocultural assumptions about how to communicate with others. Their study proposes a distinction between language differences (such as pronunciation, intonation, grammar and vocabulary) and cultural differences between patient and doctor that become manifest in patient talk. The latter refer specifically to self-presentation. Immigrant patients may present a low self-display by not saying much during interaction, or they may structure the information by first explaining the context and only at the end of the consultation indicating the main reason for the visit. There also seems to be more topic overload from these patients, i.e. more topics are introduced by them, sometimes even though the topic currently under discussion is not yet closed. Additionally, interaction may be marked by a lot of overlaps and interruptions. Based on their findings, Roberts *et al.* (2005) conclude that miscommunication in intercultural interaction is visible in communicative actions and is partly due to cultural differences (which are manifest through language). Misunderstandings may also occur due to a patient's lack of institutional knowledge, which might not be necessarily caused by their cultural background.

As communication with immigrants and patients with poor language proficiency is more problematic than with indigenous Dutch patients, the question arises as to how an interpreter can facilitate mutual understanding between doctor and patient. In the present study, the focus lies on the quality of informal interpreting in medical encounters. The issues discussed cover communication problems, the quality of interpreted talk and the dynamics of role-taking in interaction between doctor, patient and interpreter. More specifically, the discourse structures of the medical encounter are related to the level of externally assessed mutual understanding between GP and patient.

6.2 Data and method

Subjects and procedure

Analyses were based on 16 transcripts of videos derived from a dataset of the Rotterdam Intercultural Communication in the Medical Setting (RICIM) study, a project in which 430 migrant general practice patients in Rotterdam participated (Harmsen 2003; Twilt 2007). The largest group of these immigrant patients had Turkish, Surinamese, Antillean, Moroccan, Cape Verdian or eastern European backgrounds. The patients' ethnicities were based on their own and their parents' country of birth (Instituut voor Sociologisch-Economisch Onderzoek [ISEO] 1987).

In 50 of these encounters, the patient was accompanied by an informal interpreter. All GP visits were recorded on video; all patients were interviewed at home in their preferred language three to eight days after the GP consultation. Doctors filled out questionnaires regarding the specific interviews with these individual patients. All participating doctors and patients gave informed consent.

For purposes of the present study, three-party interaction involving the largest immigrant group available was selected, i.e. the Turkish group. This allowed for a more or less homogenous group, from the viewpoint of interpreter needs. Further, to optimize the comparison a selection was made based on the lowest and highest quartiles of level of mutual understanding between GP and patient (see next section), which resulted in 2 × 8 = 16 medical interviews. The interpreters were partners, family members or friends of the patients. The video data were transcribed following conversation analytical conventions (ten Have 1999), which were adapted to suit the aim of this study. In particular, Turkish elements were both transcribed in the original language and translated into Dutch. The translation was undertaken by a second-generation Turkish research assistant.

Measures

In order to answer the research questions, data were gathered on (1) level of mutual understanding between doctor and patient, externally assessed, and (2) communication elements that became apparent through reconstruction of the actual discourse (Twilt 2007). This enabled a comparison between the two levels of mutual understanding, as assessed afterwards by interviewing patient and doctor and in terms of communication processes as they unfold in the actual discourse. In other words, we compared the outcome of external criteria with the actual communicative actions via analysis of discourse (Koole and ten Thije 2000; ten Thije 2016).

External assessment of mutual understanding

The effectiveness of communication in terms of mutual understanding was measured by the Mutual Understanding Scale, which was developed and validated by a multi-ethnic and multidisciplinary expert panel using nominal group technique (Harmsen *et al.* 2005). The level of mutual understanding was calculated by comparing the information given in the interview (see above) by doctors and patients on roughly five components of the consultation: main symptom, cause of the illness, diagnosis, examination and prescribed therapy. Mutual understanding was present if both doctor and patient gave similar answers as assessed by two judges independently.

In 70% of cases there was independent agreement. All remaining cases (30%) were discussed until consensus was reached. This procedure resulted in an overall score for level of mutual understanding for each consultation on a scale between 1 (very low) and +1 (very high). For purposes of this study, consultations with scores in the lowest (between 1.0 and 0.40) and the highest (between +0.55 and +1.0) quartiles were selected. This resulted in 8 consultations with poor mutual understanding (named *low MU group*) and 8 consultations with good mutual understanding (named *high MU group*).

Analysis of discourse

The analysis of the actual discourse was performed on five communication elements related to the changes made by the interpreter in interaction. The first element refers to (1) the roles and identities of the interpreter, and we subsequently focused on (2) miscommunication and its causes and (3) the changes in the translation. Lastly, the contextual information was observed, in terms of (4) additional information and (5) side-talk activity (Twilt 2007). These elements will make clear the ways in which the interpreters engaged themselves during the interaction. Coding in accordance with the roles of facilitator, intermediary and direct source identified by Hasselkus (1992) described above was undertaken by one researcher, who was largely ignorant of the level of MU of the specific encounter. Based on the literature, one may expect there to be more miscommunication in the low MU group than in the high MU group. Also, the number of translation changes might be fewer in the high MU group.

In what follows, a description of the differences between the two groups (low MU versus high MU) is given. The main findings will be illustrated by excerpts of transcripts and detailed commentary, and structured along the five elements of the reconstruction of discourse.

6.3 Results

Roles and identities

The interpreter as facilitator (see Table 6.1, above) will mostly translate the utterances of the primary speakers literally, which corresponds to the translation-machine model (Bot 2005). As direct source role, the interpreter will probably follow the interactive model; he or she will take on an active role within the communication as a third speaker. The intermediary takes an in-between role and will not only translate, but also try to act as a mediator/culture broker during the encounter.

The role of the interpreter was assessed by identifying the number of components in every transcript. This provided insight into the way an interpreter as a third party related within the interaction and how involved he/she was with the patient. It appeared that all three roles were represented nearly equally in both groups (see Table 6.2). This suggests that the different roles do not relate to the level of mutual understanding between doctor and patient.

Table 6.2 Results for interpreter roles.

Role	Encounters with low MU	Encounters with high MU
Facilitator	3	4
Intermediary	3	3
Direct source	2	1

Upon closer observation, however, it was noticed that the role-taking was partly related to the relationship between patient and interpreter. If the partner of the patient was the interpreter, he or she could perform all roles. Other family members, like sisters and aunts, instead mostly only facilitated the interaction – and if the interpreter was the patient's son or daughter, he or she always took on the role of facilitator. This suggests that family interpreters, especially children, value understanding on a linguistic level highly. Hence the relationship between patient and interpreter seems partly to determine the role-taking. Excerpt 1 illustrates the role of facilitator. It starts with the physical exam of the patient's ear. The transcription conventions can be found in Appendix 1.

Excerpt 1: [111001] Example of facilitator role. GP = General Practitioner; IP = Interpreter; P = Patient; WF = Wife

GP: then we shall have to take a
↑lamp first
IP: (1.4) °lambasini aliyor°

(1.4)takes his lamp
GP: so ↑itch in the ears, since
a ↑long time, hh and the
medicines never helped.
IP: °(no)°=
GP: =have you been for those
symptoms (.5) have you been
to a specialist for the
symptom about the ears?
IP: eh: seye↑ gittinmi? (.)
ozel hastaneye veya ozel
bi-doktora gittinmi?
Kullagin ‘ icin
eh: have you been to thing?
have you been to a special
hospital or to a special
doctor? for your ear
P: yog↑ (0.5) yog↑
No (0.5) no
IP: No

The interpreter, who is the son of the patient, even translates the actions of the doctor that the patient is able to see for himself, like ‘takes his lamp’ (line 3), which emphasizes the importance that translating precisely has for the interpreter. In lines 5–7, the GP gives a summary of what has been discussed before, which the interpreter confirms (in line 8). In lines 13–16, the son translates the GP’s question as accurately as possible for his father. His father’s answer is translated for the GP correctly. In these instances, the son is facilitating the communication between his father and the doctor.

An example of the direct source role is given in Excerpt 2. The interpreter speaks on behalf of his wife (the patient), who barely speaks Dutch. The conversation is obviously dominated by the interpreter and the GP.

Excerpt 2: [310701] Example of direct source role

IP: (↑every time she reads)
GP: yes
IP: she has a headache [and itchy eyes
GP: [hm hm
hm hm (.9) hm (1) and when
she watches television, is
she nearby (*the screen*)? or

far away?
IP: yes, always far away
GP: yes (1.7) and what are your
concerns, that something is
wrong with her ↑head, with
something ↑else
IP: well, to be honest eh (.5)
she is concerned about the
↑eyes
GP: about the eyes themselves
IP: yes
GP: hm hm

In this excerpt, the GP's questions are directly addressed to and answered by the interpreter. The husband also expresses the concerns of his wife about her itchy eyes in lines 14–16 without addressing her first. The excerpt shows that the GP and the interpreter are talking about the patient, which is typical for the direct source role. The use of the third person ('she/her') in the conversation illustrates this even further.

Miscommunication and its causes

Miscommunication may arise from grammatical differences in language and sociocultural differences between the participants (Gass and Varonis 1991). The problems that occur may or may not be recognized, commented on or solved by the participants during the interaction. The analysis included the following categories (Gass and Varonis 1991: 139):

1. immediate recognition of the problem, with or without comment from the participant(s);
2. later recognition of the problem, with or without comment from the participant(s);
3. no recognition of the problem.

Excerpt 3 illustrates an immediate recognition of the problem.

Excerpt 3: [101808] Example of immediate recognition

IP: no for him eh (avkat)
(*lawyer*)
P: °avkat°
lawyer

5 GP: ↑eye doctor?
6 P: avkat
7 *lawyer*
8 IP: avkat
9 *lawyer*
10 GP: (.5) 'augat' ((tries to
11 repeat the interpreter))
12 P: yes
13 IP: yes
14 GP: wait, <I don't understand>,
15 what (.) what is 'augat'?
((interruption by phone call GP))
27 IP: for the 'augat' here ↑this
28 ((points to form of patient))
29 GP: 'augat' ((looks at form))
30 °what is this then° (.4)
31 oh, '<↑lawyer>', [sorry,
32 now I understand
33 IP: [yes, 'lawyer'
34 GP: finally, '↑lawyer'
35 IP: yes

The problem in this excerpt is that the GP does not understand the word 'avkat' or 'aukat' (lines 1–13). In lines 14–15, we see that the problem is immediately recognized by the GP when he explicitly comments 'I don't understand, what is "augat"?'. A resolution is attempted after discussing about the communication problem, subsequently leading to the correct understanding by the GP ('"lawyer", now I understand' – lines 30–32), which is acknowledged by the interpreter (lines 33 and 35). An example of later recognition of the problem will be given later in this section.

When no recognition takes place, it means that only an observer after the interaction recognizes the misunderstanding. Such misunderstandings can become transparent during discourse analysis (see also Meeuwesen *et al.* 2010). To assess the possible causes of these communication problems, we used the categorisation of Roberts *et al.* (2005: 39ff), who analysed intercultural interactions between family physicians and patients in London, identifying four main causes of miscommunication:

1. *Pronunciation*: the wrong pronunciation of words and sentences can lead to misunderstanding between participants;
2. *Intonation*: problems occur because of unexpected intonation, rhythm and melody in the official language;

3. *Grammar and vocabulary*: flawed use of grammar rules, vocabulary, time markers and sentence construction can lead to misunderstanding between the participants; and
4. *Style of self-presentation*: features of this category are self-profile, information-structuring style, topic overload and overlapping speech. The ways in which the speaker presents himself through his language use may lead to misunderstanding between the participants. These ways are often culturally determined.

Applying these two category systems enables detection of types and causes of miscommunication, and the ways in which the participants react to this.

Table 6.3 shows that the low MU group contained far more cases of miscommunication (83% versus 17%). On three occasions (all in the low MU group) the problems were not recognized by the participants (and therefore were not solved). All examples of miscommunication in the high MU group were recognized by the participants.

Table 6.3 Number of communication problems in 16 encounters, comparing groups with low and high mutual understanding (MU) between doctor and patient.

Communication problems	Low MU (n = 8)	High MU (n = 8)
Immediate recognition of the problem, with or without comment	6	1
Later recognition of the problem, with or without comment	6	2
No recognition of the problem	3	–
Total	15 (83%)	3 (17%)

Excerpt 4 shows an example of a communication problem that came up, which was later recognized and eventually solved. The cause of the communication problem lies in the lack of Dutch vocabulary of the interpreter, who is the son of the patient.

Excerpt 4: [111001] Communication problem, later recognized

GP: have you ever had an ear
↑lavage?

IP: simdi sey varmi?
intablanma? disariya dogru
pislik?
now is there thing? an
infection? dirt to the
outside?
P: bazi icinde var pislik,
bazi kasin t-
there is some dirty
inside(the ear), that itch-
IP: yok yani (.) sey olarak
su gibi cikan pislik
no mean (.) just like
thing dirty that it goes
out like water

In lines 97–98 the GP asks if the patient has ever had an ear lavage before. In lines 99–101 the interpreter translates 'an ear lavage' as 'an infection'. Because of the lack of (medical) vocabulary of the interpreter, miscommunication occurs between the patient and the GP. As Excerpt 5 shows, the problem was solved later in the encounter.

Excerpt 5: [111001] Communication problem, later recognized and solved

P: gondersin kulak doktorunada,
burada bir yikama yapti.
O yikamada biraz fayda '
[buldum biliyonmu?!
let him send to an ear
specialist, but he had it
washed out here once
(the ear). During that
rinse I found some help, '
you know?
GP: [and for that
IP: Eh: he says that eh before
eh what eh clean eh made
eh: his ↑ears,
GP: yes
IP: after that clean eh: made
some, ↑some went better
GP: and just ↑now I asked if I
cleaned it and I believe you
said no then (.) d- you z-
didn't I just ask you if it

was washed out here?
IP: you didn't ask me that.
GP: yes: yes I did ask if it
was washed ↑out you said if
it was washed with water
IP: *yes*
GP: I heard you translate it

As the patient says that he had received an ear lavage once (lines 269–272), the GP now makes the problem visible (lines 286–290) by combining this information with his question earlier in the conversation ('and just now I asked if I cleaned it and I believe you said no then'). The GP then discusses with the interpreter what went wrong before in the translation process.

The majority of these communication problems occurred due to the style of self-presentation (Table 6.4), where the interpreter showed a low self-profile, e.g. by having difficulties in structuring the information given by the patient. Other causes were inability to pronounce words or form words or sentences in the Dutch language correctly.

Table 6.4 Causes of communication problems.

Causes	Low MU	High MU	Total
Pronunciation	4	–	4 (24%)
Intonation	–	–	–
Grammar and vocabulary	4	1	5 (29%)
Style of self-presentation	7	2	9 (47%)

These excerpts show that communication problems may occur because of a wrong translation and/or the interpreter's lack of (medical) vocabulary in Dutch. The excerpts also show the ways in which such communication problems are later recognized and resolved.

Changes in translation

The translations being rendered by the interpreter were analysed on a global level in terms of the content changes that occurred in translation, as derived from Aranguri *et al.* (2006: 626):

1. *Content revisions*: the interpreter changes the content of the translation by altering important information;

2. *Content omissions*: the interpreter leaves out important information while translating; and
3. *Content reductions*: the interpreter reduces the content of the utterance of the primary speaker. In this category the interpreter synthesizes the utterances of the speaker, mostly following after a long utterance of the primary speaker.

The authors indicate that these categories are not mutually exclusive, in that e.g. revision also implies omission. However, these changes in translation give a rough indication of the quality of the translation – revisions and omissions may be serious flaws in the translation, while content reductions seem more or less acceptable.

Table 6.5 shows that the low MU group contained twice as many content changes in translation than the high MU group (65% versus 35%). Content omissions, leaving out important information, happened most frequently (48% of both groups).

Table 6.5 Changes in translation.

Changes	Low MU	High MU	Total
Content revisions	11	8	19 (32%)
Content omissions	21	8	29 (48%)
Content reductions	7	5	12 (20%)
Total	39 (65%)	21 (35%)	60 (100%)

Excerpt 6 shows an example of a content omission. During this encounter a married couple visits the GP and their daughter functions as the interpreter. The patient is trying to explain his complaint – he has a painful, purple foot. His partner (wife) also joins the discussion. Early in the encounter the patient tells the story that he stood on something, which may have caused the painful foot.

Excerpt 6: [310714] Example of content omission

P: surdan soyleydi [( ) ben
birseye bastiydim
from here it was so [( )
I pressed on something
(= stood)
IP: and then over here)

WF: [bastim deme sus bir kontrol
etsin
[don't say I stood (on
something). quiet, let her
check
GP: [yes °well° it isn't purple
↑now, fortunately
IP: no ↑ not that
GP: no

In lines 876–877 the patient points out where the foot was purple, and this is when he says that he stood on something. The interpreter translates the part 'and then over here' (line 881), but leaves out the part where the patient mentioned that he had stood on something. The patient's wife comments on the request of the patient in lines 882–883. She directs him not to mention the incident and to wait for the GP to look at the foot. Both the wife and the interpreter may think that this request has nothing to do with the complaint, but it is up to the GP to decide. However, this seems important for the patient, because prior to this excerpt he also had mentioned this request. The GP did not receive this information during the encounter either.

A greater number of linguistic problems occur in the low MU group, because the interpreters' language proficiency appears to be inadequate. Changes in translation, especially omissions, may lead to a decrease in mutual understanding between the GP and the patient during the discourse. As already seen, the majority of the communication problems can be related to the style of self-presentation.

Additional information

Additional information consists of the interpreter's supply of knowledge beyond the actual information given by the patient or the GP in the encounter. We distinguish between background information and small talk. The presence of small talk in medical encounters stimulates communication between the participants (Aranguri *et al.* 2006) and gives information about their relationship. Background information, meanwhile, is information given by the interpreter about the patient, that is not initiated by the patient but by the interpreter. This is not something that distinguishes a formal interpreter from an informal interpreter (Rosenberg *et al.* 2007), and it may reflect caregiver role-taking by an informal interpreter.

Table 6.6 Kinds of additional information.

Additional information	Encounters with low MU	Encounters with high MU
Background	35	6
Small talk	5	5
Total	40	11

Table 6.6 shows that six times as much background information is provided in the low MU group than in the high MU group. For small talk, there were no differences between the two groups.

The large amount of additional information provided in the group with low mutual understanding can be seen as evidence of the interpreter's effort. As this happens mostly where there is poor mutual understanding between patient and doctor, one may speculate that the interpreter complicates the communication with this information overload. Thus, background information provided on by an informal interpreter seems to be not very effective.

An example of providing this background information is given in Excerpt 7. In this extract the interpreter (who is a friend of the patient) mentions the concerns of the patient. The latter does not mention these feelings herself. The dialogue is between the interpreter and the GP.

Excerpt 7: [200309] Example of giving background information

1 IP: she be scared, eh maybe
2 becomes ↑asthma
3 GP: [yes
4 IP: [I do ↑not think, but eh
5 she be sca[red
6 GP: [she she is scared of that
7 IP: yes scared

The interpreter and the GP are talking about chest problems of the patient's baby. The interpreter says in lines 1–2 that she thinks the patient is scared of her child having asthma. This information about the feelings of the patient is not checked by the interpreter or by the GP with the patient. The GP seems to rely on the additional information provided by the informal interpreter.

Side-talk activity

The presence of side-talk activity (Wadensjö 1998) says something about the interpreter's degree of control during interaction, because he or she can initiate, maintain or stop the communication activity. The elements of the transcripts in which at least two turns of the interpreter as well as the patient followed subsequently without interruption by the GP were counted as side-talk activity.

Instances of side-talk activity happened twice as often in the low MU group (17, versus 8 in the high MU group). Most of the side talk occurred between the patient and the interpreter, which resulted in exclusion of the GP from the interaction. The frequent occurrence of side talk seems to complicate the interaction between the GP and the patient. The interpreter explains and talks more to the patient, to make the GP's contribution more understandable, but in fact this seems to have an adverse effect, evidenced in a lower level of mutual understanding.

Moreover, side-talk activity was mostly found in consultations in which more than three persons participated (family members or friends of the patient). Excerpt 8 illustrates side-talk activity in a consultation involving four participants: the GP, the patient, his wife and the interpreter. It begins with the interpreter translating the advice of the (female) GP.

Excerpt 8: [310714] Example of side-talk

IP: if it happens again, she
says, take it with you, we
can have a look, she says,
now nothing she says
P: su gozumde sey var
on this eye, there is
thing
suramda
here ((points at one of
his eyes))
WF: ne var?
what is there?
P: birsey yok!
there is nothing!
WF: niye kahirleniyorsunki?
why are you getting
irritated?
IP: ne var, de
what is the matter, say it

WF: [suralari soyle sisiyorya
(.) onu sey ediyor
here and there it becomes
so big (.) that thing he
does
((points at the patients
face))
P: [sura
here
WF: surda bak, biricik birsey
gibi
here look, just like thing
IP: from the inside, he has this
bump

In line 5 the patient brings up a new complaint about his eye. The interpreter discusses this with the patient and his wife without informing the GP (line 3 through line 31). The complaint seems to be clearer after this discussion, but the GP only receives a minimum of information from the interpreter in lines 32–33 ('from the inside, he has this bump'). The GP can only speculate what was communicated between the interpreter, the patient and his wife.

6.4 Discussion

The findings of this study lead us to formulate a number of conclusions and some critical comments. First, the subsequent external assessment of mutual understanding between doctor and patient corresponds fairly well with the level of miscommunication in the actual medical encounters that were analysed via the five elements of communication in this study. As anticipated, there were more instances of miscommunication in the low MU group than in the high MU group. The causes for such miscommunication were mainly due to the interpreters' low-profile presentation (e.g. hesitations, problems in structuring information). The omissions of content occurred most frequently in the translation process, which is in line with the findings of Aranguri *et al.* (2006) findings. These are also consistent with findings from the hospital setting (Pöchhhacker 2007; Wolffers *et al.* 2007).

Furthermore, frequent conveyance of background information by the interpreter as well as side talk (between the interpreter and the patient) appears to make it difficult for the doctor to follow the interaction, as well as for the interpreter to coordinate it. This happened mostly in the low MU group. It turns out that the informal interpreter generally takes on a central role in the communication process by giving background information about the patient and in trying to control and coordinate the encounter. The interpreter forms the essential link in the intercultural constellation of the medical encounter. Informal interpreters are thus active participants performing multiple roles. These findings confirm present theories of interpreting (Wadensjö 1998; Bolden 2000; Bot 2005; Rosenberg *et al.* 2007; Evrin and Meyer 2016), which claim that interpreters are not just translation machines but have an active role in the interaction. We have seen that these roles cover more than translating alone, but also aspects of being an advocate of the patient. Young interpreters do value the linguistic understanding between patient and doctor. This is consistent with findings of Green *et al.* (2005) that young interpreters see medical translating for their family as a serious and very responsible task. At the same time, as we saw, informal interpreters differ from each other in their role performance, and this may either facilitate or hinder the medical encounter. An interpreter performing the role of a direct source is most likely to hinder the communication, by giving background information, and by frequently engaging in side talk. These issues have been indicated by physicians as difficulties when confronted with a patient and an informal interpreter: they wonder what the patient and family interpreter are discussing together, especially if they receive brief bits of information after a long stretch of side talk. When family interpreters in the role of caregivers become the direct source, this is particularly ineffective (cf. Hasselkus 1992; Rosenberg *et al.* 2008).

Some methodological remarks are in order. This study was not intended to generalize regarding the quality of informal interpreting. Instead, the small research sample (n = 16) provided a rich understanding of relevant interactional mechanisms in the process of exploring the quality of informal interpreting. Also, by applying several observation techniques (analysing five elements of communication) to describe the actual discourse – techniques which all more or less pointed in the same direction in terms of differences between low and high MU groups – the study reaches accountable reliability. Furthermore, the coding was performed blind, which also contributes to the reliability. The comparison of an external assessment of mutual understanding (based on participants' statements) with the observations of actual discourse contributes to the validity of the assessments. The detailed analysis offered useful insight into what actually happens in the interaction, including which elements cause misunderstanding.

Only Turkish-speaking interpreters participated in this study. It remains to be seen to what extent the findings would be applicable to other migrant patient groups, although it is likely that the results will be valid where the patient variables – education, Dutch language proficiency, cultural views – are similar. Nevertheless, it would be interesting to conduct further research in which different migrant groups are compared with each other. It is recommended that similar research be undertaken with larger groups and with patients from different origins, and further comparisons made between informal and formal interpreters. In general, more research based on the discourse analysis of informal interpreting is needed.

Researchers on interpreters' work in health care are often keen to recommend the use of formal or professional interpreters. However, such studies are often limited to interviews or surveys (Flores 2005; Jacobs *et al.* 2006). Observational and sociolinguistic studies focused on the actual communicative actions of interpreters are scarce; exceptions include studies by Aranguri *et al.* (2006) and Bührig and Meyer (2004), who analysed authentic data of informal interpreting in hospitals within a discourse analytical approach (see also Evrin and Meyer 2016). Attitudes towards the use of informal interpreters are mainly negative, even without conclusive research. However, despite the evidence of problems with informal interpreting, it is clear that the use of informal interpreters can sometimes substantially facilitate medical communication (Meeuwesen *et al.* 2010).

Appendix: Transcription conventions

italics	English translation of Turkish utterances
	upward intonation
word	stressed word
<slow>	slow tempo
°low°	low volume
e::::h	indicates stretching of sounds it follows
'h'	spoken with laughter
wo-	abortion of utterance
hh.	in-breath audible inspiration

(.)	pause, below 0.3 seconds
(0.4)(1,0)	pause of 0.4 and 1.0 seconds
((text))	commentary from the researcher
(xxx)	incomprehensible
[	overlapping utterances
	wo [rd
	[word
=	latching
	word =
	=word

References

Apfelbaum, Birgit (1998) 'I think I have to translate first...': Zu Problemen der Gesprächsorganisation in Dolmetchensituationen sowie zu einigen interaktiven Verfahren ihrer Bearbeitung. In Birgit Apfelbaum and Hermann Müller (eds) *Fremde in Gespräch: Gesprächsanalytische Untersuchungen zu Dolmetsch, Interaktionen, Interkultureller Kommunikation und institutionalisierten Interaktionsformen*, 21–46. Frankfurt: IKO-Verlag fur interkulturelle Kommunikation.

Aranguri, Cesar, Brad Davidson and Robert Ramirez (2006) Patterns of communication through interpreters: A detailed sociolinguistic analysis. *Journal of General Internal Medicine* 21 (6): 623–629. https://doi.org/10.1111/j.1525-1497.2006.00451.x

Baraldi, Claudio and Laura Gavioli (2016) On professional and non-professional interpreting in healthcare services: The case of intercultural mediators. *European Journal of Applied Linguistics* 4 (1): 33–55. https://doi.org/10.1515/eujal-2015-0026

Bolden, Galina B. (2000) Toward understanding practices of medical interpreting: Interpreters' involvement in history taking. *Discourse Studies* 2 (4): 387–419. https://doi.org/10.1177/1461445600002004001

Bot, Hanneke (2005) *Dialogue Interpreting in Mental Health*. Amsterdam: Rodopi.

Bührig, Kristin, Juliane House and Jan ten Thije (eds) (2009) *Translatory Action and Intercultural Communication*. Manchester: St. Jerome.

Bührig, Kristin and Bernd Meyer (2004) *Ad hoc*-interpreting and the achievement of communicative purposes in doctor-patient-communication. In J. House and J. Rehbein (eds) *Multilingual Communication*, 43–62. Amsterdam: Benjamins. https://doi.org/10.1075/hsm.3.04buh

Bührig, Kristin and Jochen Rehbein (1996) *Reproduzierendes Handeln: Ubersetzen, Simultanes und Konsekutieves Dolmetschen im Diskurs-analytischen Vergleich.* Hamburg: Arbeiten zur Mehrsprachigkeit.

Centraal Bureau voor de Statistiek (CBS) (2015) Statline. Available online: http://statline.cbs.nl/

Evrin, Feyza and Bernd Meyer (ed) (2016) *Non-Professional Interpreting and Translation: Translational Cultures in Focus.* Special Issue of *European Journal of Applied Linguistics* 4 (1). https://doi.org/10.1515/eujal-2015-0042

Flores, Glenn (2005) The impact of medical interpreter services on the quality of health care: A systematic review. *Medical Care Research and Review* 62 (2): 255–299. https://doi.org/10.1177/1077558705275416

Gass, Susan M. and Evangeline M. Varonis (1991) Miscommunication in nonnative speaker discourse. In Nikolas Coupland, Howard Giles and John M. Wiemann (eds) *'Miscommunication' and Problematic Talk*, 121–145. Newbury Park, CA: Sage.

Green, Judith, Caroline Free, Vanita Bhavnani and Tony Newman (2004) Translators and mediators: Bilingual young people's accounts of their interpreting work in health care. *Social Science and Medicine* 60 (9): 2097–2110. https://doi.org/10.1016/j.socscimed.2004.08.067

Harmsen, J. A. M. [Hans] (2003) *When Cultures Meet in Medical Practice: Improvement in Intercultural Communication Evaluated.* Rotterdam: Erasmus Universiteit Rotterdam.

Harmsen, J. A. M. [Hans], Roos M. D. Bernsen, Ludwien Meeuwesen, David Pinto and Marc A. Bruijnzeels (2005) Assessment of mutual understanding of physician patient encounters: Development and validation of a mutual understanding scale (MUS) in a multicultural general practice setting. *Patient Education and Counseling* 59 (2): 171–181. https://doi.org/10.1016/j.pec.2004.11.003

Hasselkus, Betty R. (1992) The family caregiver as interpreter in the geriatric medical interview. *Medical Anthropology Quarterly* (New Series) 6 (3): 288–304. https://doi.org/10.1525/maq.1992.6.3.02a00070

Instituut voor Sociologisch-Economisch Onderzoek (ISEO) (1987) *Beter Meten 1.* [Better measurements 1]. Rotterdam: Instituut voor Sociaal Economisch Onderzoek.

Jacobs, Elizabeth, Alice Hm Chen, Leah S. Karliner, Niels Agger-Gupta and Sunita Mutha (2006) The need for more research on language barriers in health care: A proposed research agenda. *The Milbank Quarterly* 84 (1): 111–133. https://doi.org/10.1111/j.1468-0009.2006.00440.x

Kleinman, Arthur M. (1980) *Patients and Healers in the Context of Culture.* Berkeley: University of California Press.

Knapp-Potthoff, Annelie and Karlfried Knapp (1986) Interweaving two discourses – The difficult task of the non-professional interpreter. In Juliane House and Shoshana (eds) *Interlingual and Intercultural Communication: Discourse and Cognition in Translation and Second Language Acquisition Studies*, 151–169. Tübingen: Narr.

Knapp-Potthoff, Annelie and Karlfried Knapp (1987) The man or woman in the middle: Discoursal aspects of non-professional interpreting. In Karlfried Knapp, Werner Enninger and Annelie Knapp-Potthoff (eds) *Analyzing Intercultural Communication*. Studies in Anthropological Linguistics 1: 181–212. Berlin: De Gruyter. https://doi.org/10.1515/9783110874280

Koole, Tom and Jan D. ten Thije (2000) The reconstruction of intercultural discourse: Methodological considerations. *Journal of Pragmatics* 33 (4): 571–587. https://doi.org/10.1016/S0378-2166(00)00035-7

Meeuwesen, Ludwien, J. A. M. [Hans] Harmsen, Roos M. D. Bernsen and Marc A. Bruijnzeels (2006) Do Dutch doctors communicate differently with immigrant patients than with Dutch patients? *Social Science and Medicine* 63 (9): 2407–2417. https://doi.org/10.1016/j.socscimed.2006.06.005

Meeuwesen, Ludwien, Sione Twilt, Jan D. ten Thije and Hans Harmsen (2010) 'Ne diyor?' (What does she say?): Informal interpreting in general practice. *Patient Education and Counseling* 81 (2): 198–203. https://doi.org/10.1016/j.pec.2009.10.005

Pöchhacker, Franz (2007) *Dolmetschen: Konzeptuelle Grundlagen und Deskriptive Untersuchungen.* Tübungen: Stauffenberg.

Robb, Nadia and Trisha Greenhalgh (2005) 'You have to cover up the words of the doctor': The mediation of trust in interpreted consultations in primary care. *Journal of Health Organization and Management* 20 (5): 434–455. https://doi.org/10.1108/14777260610701803

Roberts, Celia, Becky Moss, Val Wass, Srikant Sarangi and Roger Jones (2005) Misunderstandings: A qualitative study of primary care consultations in multilingual settings, and educational implications. *Medical Education* 39 (5): 465–475. https://doi.org/10.1111/j.1365-2929.2005.02121.x

Rosenberg, Ellen, Yvan Leanza and Robbyn Seller (2007) Doctor-patient communication in primary care with an interpreter: Physician perceptions of professional and family interpreters. *Patient Education and Counseling* 67 (3): 286–292. https://doi.org/10.1016/j.pec.2007.03.011

Rosenberg, Ellen, Robbyn Seller and Yvan Leanza (2008) Through interpreters' eyes: Comparing roles of professional and family interpreters. *Patient Education and Counseling* 70 (1): 87–93. https://doi.org/10.1016/j.pec.2007.09.015

ten Have, Paul (1999) *Doing Conversation Analysis.* London: Sage.

ten Thije, Jan D. (2009) The self-retreat of the interpreter: An analysis of teasing and toasting in intercultural discourse. In Kristin Bührig, Juliane House and Jan ten Thije (eds) *Translatory Action and Intercultural Communication*, 114–155. Manchester: St. Jerome.

ten Thije, Jan D. (2016) Intercultural communication. In Ludwig Jäger, Werner Holly, Peter Krapp, Samuel Weber and Simone Heekeren (eds) *Ein internationales Handbuch zu Linguistik als Kulturwissenschaft / An International Handbook of Linguistics as a Cultural Discipline*. Handbuch zu Linguistik als Kulturwissenschaft 43: 582–593. Berlin: Mouton de Gruyter.

Twilt, Sione (2007) *'Hmm... hoe zal ik dat vertellen?': De rol van de niet professionele tolk in arts-patiënt gesprekken*. Unpublished master's dissertation, Utrecht University, Utrecht.

Wadensjö, Cecilia (1998) *Interpreting as Interaction*. Harlow, UK: Addison Wesley Longman.

Wolffers, Ivan, Bart Wolf, Hetty van den Oever, Fedde Scheele, Marianne van Elteren, Kathleen Welborn and Marius Leest (2007) Zorgverleners cultureel competent? Noodzaak van culturele competenties in de omgang met patiënten in ziekenhuizen [Are health care providers culturally competent?]. *Cultuur Migratie Gezondheid* 4 (2): 78–86

Zendedel, Rena (2017) *Informal Interpreting in Dutch General Practice*. Unpublished doctoral dissertation. University of Amsterdam: Amsterdam.

Sione Twilt wrote her master's thesis on the discourse of informal interpreting in general practice. She was involved in the European Grundtvig project 'TRICC' as a coordinator and researcher (www.tricc-eu.net) and currently teaches healthcare students in Rotterdam. Furthermore she is currently involved in analysing professional interactions between Dutch-speaking speech and language therapists and multilingual clients. Address for correspondence: Rotterdam University of Applied Sciences, School of Healthcare, Rochussentraat 198, 3015 EK, Rotterdam, The Netherlands.
Email: s.twilt@hr.nl

Ludwien Meeuwesen was associate professor at the Department of Interdisciplinary Social Science at Utrecht University. She was actively involved in research and projects concerning medical communication, specifically migrant health, until shortly before her sudden death.

Jan D. ten Thije is Associate Professor at the Department of Languages, Literature and Communication at Utrecht University. He coordinates the master's programme in Intercultural Communication and the Intercultural

Competence project. His main fields of research concern institutional discourse in multicultural and international settings, *lingua receptiva* / receptive multilingualism, intercultural training, language education and functional pragmatics. Address for correspondence: Trans 10, 3512 JK Utrecht, The Netherlands.
Email: j.d.tenthije@uu.nl

Hans Harmsen worked as a general practitioner in a multicultural neighbourhood in Rotterdam from 1980 until his retirement. As a trainer of GPs he was allied with the Department of General Practice of the Erasmus MC, Rotterdam. In 2003 he obtained his PhD, with his thesis titled *When Culture Meets in General Practice: Improvement in Intercultural Communication Evaluated.*

7 Third party insurance?: Interactional role alignment in family member mediated primary care consultations

Celia Roberts & Srikant Sarangi

7.1 Introduction

The insurance industry in most countries offers 'third party' insurance to protect those who are found to be responsible if a claim is made against them. In healthcare encounters, the third party represents a rather different kind of insurance. Although family members may be seen as to some extent the outsider in a medical transaction, as the term 'third party' suggests, they help to mediate the encounter in highly significant ways. In this regard, the role-responsibilities of the doctor, the family member and the patient are likely to shift during the triadic encounter, producing more complex participant frameworks (Goffman 1981) which affect the communicative environment.

Intercultural healthcare encounters are a routine feature of healthcare delivery (Schouten and Meeuwesen 2006; Sarangi 2012), typical of the 'superdiversity' of globalized communities (Vertovec 2007, 2010). The extent to which trained interpreters can insure the consultation against misunderstandings and unspoken agendas has been the subject of much research and debate. Of equal interest, however, has been how a third-party presence can lead to misunderstandings based on inaccurate relay of words and ideas. Most of the literature has assumed that triadic consultations are interpreter-mediated and the focus has been on linguistic aspects as well as interactional aspects of the encounter. However, mediated interactions with a third-party non-interpreter presence are common in the healthcare setting. For instance, the parent in a paediatric encounter and a spouse or offspring in a geriatric encounter do not attend the clinic in the primary role as interpreter and/or mediator but as carer, although they may be drawn into the communicative activities of mediation and interpretation in a given encounter.

In this paper we examine two encounters where family members are present. Both of the encounters are mediated, in that the companion becomes involved in the interaction from an early stage and this leads to a three-way conversation in which the third party takes on the role of making talk (more) understandable and of contributing to managing the doctor–patient relationship. While the literature on interpreting addresses a wide range of definitions for these triadic encounters, we will use the term 'companion' for the first case, which is a monolingual encounter in English, and the term 'lay interpreter' (or family interpreter as they are widely known in the UK) for the second case, where the daughter interprets for her Turkish-speaking mother but has no training as an interpreter.

We proceed as follows. In Section 2, we review relevant studies addressing the role of the interpreter. This is followed, in Section 3, by an outlining of our data corpus and methodology, including the choice of an analytical framework to engage with the empirical data. In Section 4, we offer in-depth analysis of the two encounters. Section 5 provides a discussion of the key findings, where mediation in triadic settings is conceptualized on a continuum from the most institutionalized to the most familial and personal. Section 6 offers the conclusion.

7.2 Literature review

The literature on interpreting in healthcare journals tends to be structured around two debates. The first concerns whether the interpreter should be an impartial conduit through which two languages flow or, alternatively, act as an advocate who is on the patient's side, taking up a strategic position and arguing their case (Greenhalgh *et al.* 2006; Robb and Greenhalgh 2006). The second debate is around the issue of professional versus lay interpreters, where the argument is as much about affordable financial resources for the recruitment of trained professional interpreters as about the quality of the interpreting activity itself.

The two debates are often conflated, on the assumption that an ideal model of communication is an unproblematic transmission of a message and that professional interpreters are best placed to produce this. The argument about the interpreter as a neutral tool or 'walking bilingual dictionary' (Ebden *et al.* 1988) stems from a long history of research and training that relates to conference interpreting in which linguistic accuracy, completeness and objectivity are the trademarks of the profession. While acknowledging the necessity of these standards in community and public service interpreting, Corsellis (2008) and Hale (2004) recognize that interpreting in healthcare settings is not simply a matter of the impartial transmission of accurately translated information (see also Angelelli 2005). In these settings, asymmetries of power and knowledge are compounded by complex socio-psychological dimensions such as differing cultural assumptions and levels of trust (Robb and Greenhalgh 2006), that require a more active role of the interpreter as an advocate or ambassador representing the patient (Haffner 1992) or as an intercultural mediator and co-therapist (Singy and Guex 2005). A number of studies (e.g. Wadensjö 1998; Bolden 2000; Davidson 2000; Pöchhacker 2004; Baraldi and Gavioli 2012; Raymond 2014a, 2014b; Li 2015) have focused on participant structure at the micro-interactional level without necessarily addressing issues of trust or advocacy.

The main concern in the healthcare sector in the UK has been the relative value of professional versus lay interpreters. Government and medical council policies on the use of professional interpreters vary across countries. In the UK, the official advice from the General Medical Council (GMC) is that every patient who is in need should have access to a professional interpreter. But, increasingly, the cost of such provision is part of a wider, negative debate about immigration and its financial and social costs.

In reality, most interpreter-mediated consultations in the primary care setting are with lay interpreters, usually family members (and so are often referred to as family interpreters). The extent to which such triadic encounters are successful has not been widely researched (but see Cordella 2011; Meyer 2012), although in the healthcare literature they have long been generally assumed to be problematic (Putsch 1985; Cohen *et al.* 1999). However, a few studies based on interviews and focus groups suggest that there are benefits to using family interpreters. The involvement of another family member – even if it is a child, as in the case of the study by Green *et al.* (2005) – brings intimate knowledge of the patient and emotional and interactional support to counter feelings of mistrust towards the institution of medicine and, on occasions, the professional interpreter.

Just as there has been little research on family members as interpreters, there is also little attention paid to the role of the family member as mediator as well as companion in monolingual encounters. And, indeed, these two areas of interest have not been compared systematically. Studies of consultations with family members as third parties have looked at the elderly (e.g. Coupland and Coupland 2000; Tsai 2007), at children (e.g. Tannen and Wallat 1983) and at adolescents (e.g. Silverman 1987). The issue of autonomy in both geriatric and paediatric settings comes to the fore in the interactional sense: in a seminal study, Silverman (1987) proposed the metaphor of 'chauffeuring' to describe parental involvement in the discussion and/or resolution of sensitive issues concerning diabetes management of adolescent children.

Rather than seeing interpreter-mediated consultations and non-interpreter mediated consultations as separate phenomena, it is possible to see a continuum of roles and relationships across a spectrum, with the professional interpreter as gatekeeper (Davidson 2000) at one extreme, orientating towards medical norms (Bolden 2000), and the more strategically positioned 'chauffeur' at the other, personally involved in driving the interaction to its destination. Real-life consultations, however, are always characterized by role shifts along this continuum, as we will show in the data analysis section.

7.3 Data and methodology

The data for this paper are drawn from a London-based project: Patients with Limited English and Doctors in General Practice: Educational Issues (PLEDGE) (Roberts *et al.* 2004; Moss and Roberts 2005). Although the focus of the PLEDGE project was on how patients and doctors manage the consultation in English, inevitably, the data included a sub-set of patients whose relatives or friends acted as mediators in either monolingual or multilingual encounters. Of the 232 videos recorded for the PLEDGE project, just under a quarter were with a third party. And this is certainly an under-representation, since encounters with professional interpreters or triadic encounters where virtually all the talk was not in English were not recorded. Half of the recorded triadic encounters were between parents and their babies/children and the general practitioner (GP), and most of the remainder were with elderly people who were accompanied by younger relatives as carers, mediators or 'chauffeurs'. So, although the consultation, certainly in the Western world, is normally thought of as a two-party encounter, a three-way consultation is absolutely routine (Cordella 2011; Swinglehurst *et al.* 2014).

All video recordings were viewed independently, three times, by two discourse analysts in order to screen for language and communication issues such as apparent miscommunication, repositioning of interactional alignments and so forth, and the GPs involved were asked for extended feedback on key video footage. Two pieces of data will be analysed in detail, one of a (non-interpreter-) mediated consultation with an elderly Cypriot woman who is a fluent English speaker and her daughter. The other is with a middle-aged Turkish woman and her daughter, who acts as a lay interpreter as the patient displays no knowledge of English.

Analytical framework

Our analytical framework is informed primarily by Goffman's (1983) notion of the interaction order, in particular the concepts of 'interactional frame', 'participant framework' and '(mis)alignment'. 'Frame' (Goffman 1974) is a set of understandings and assumptions relating to structure of participation based on what is going on at any particular moment in talk, while 'participant framework' (Goffman 1981) is a multiplicity of speaking and listening roles which may be operative at any given point in a social encounter. 'Alignment' (Goffman 1974) points to how an individual's contribution is in line with the other participants in the interaction. Misalignment comes about when there are discrepancies between 'what is actually taking place in a given situation and what is thought to be typical, normatively expected, probable, desirable or, in other respects, more in accord with what is culturally normal' (Stokes and Hewitt 1976: 841–842). During interactions, changes in alignment imply changes in frame, with speaker and listener roles being in constant flux. Especially in three-way communication, the roles of listener and speaker can become complicated: which hearer is the 'ratified' one?, and is the speaker 'animating' someone else's talk or are they, in Goffman's (1981) terms, the principal or author? Beyond the interaction order, these questions can have social and ethical consequences, for example when the family member is speaking to the doctor, turning the patient into a bystander or when the conversation between patient and mediator drives the interaction into a new and more emotional environment not routinely ratified in GP consultations.

Aspects of narrative theory are also drawn on in the analysis. All three participants are actively co-authoring the story of the patient, but we look here particularly at the ways in which the patient and the third party co-narrate, drawing on elements of the classic Labovian fully-fledged story structure (Labov and Waletzky 1967) and on 'small stories' (Bamberg and Georgakopoulou 2008), the fleeting, interactionally acomplished fragments of a given story.

7.4 Data analysis

The mediated consultation in English

Mrs S is an elderly Greek Cypriot woman who has a history of heart problems (with pain in her chest) and has come to the surgery, accompanied by her middle-aged daughter. She had been admitted to hospital the previous week but tests showed that she had not had another heart attack. The doctor in the video is highly experienced and, anecdotally, popular with patients. He is not the one she usually sees, so in Example 1 he has to quickly familiarize himself with her history and home situation. (Transcription conventions are provided in the Appendix.)

Example 1: D = Doctor, P = Patient, R = Patient's daughter

01 D: so how have you been
(1.0)
02 P: I've been (.) in hospital
03 D: mm
04 P: for (. .) Monday I went in on Monday and I came out
05 R: last Monday yeah sh- she
06 P: I came out Tuesday didn't I
07 R: she had chest pains an- and she came down here and they sent for an ambulance an-
08 P: and sent an ambulance from here an' [took me]
09 R: [took her]
10 P: to hospital
(. .)
11 P: then I had all these (.) tests
12 D: mm hm
13 P: injections (.) was (. .) [then they]
14 R: [and they said]

15 P: sent me home
16 R: the following day
17 P: and today I feel= =
18 R: = =she doesn't- she doesn't feel
19 P: no' alright today
20 D: what's- what's happened
21 P: s- since this morning y'know I feel my heart is (1.0) it's got this= =
22 R: = =it's not a chest pain it's like (.) it's like a murmur-y feeling

In this opening, symptom presentation and history-taking phase, the daughter's role as co-narrator is established. The patient starts the story *in media res* in turn 3, 'I've been in hospital', taking the most dramatic moment, for her, of the events of the previous week. The daughter first clarifies the time reference in turn 6, 'last Monday yeah', and also in turn 19, 'the following day', and she uses this first entry to put herself in the frame of co-narrator throughout this early stage of the consultation. She provides situational detail (turns 8–9) in the classic Labovian narrative style (Labov and Waletzky 1967) and she latches onto her mother's evaluation at turn 20 to reinforce the evaluative narrative stage of this 'small story' (Bamberg and Georgakopoulou 2008). She also tries to bring a more institutional perspective into the narrative when at turn 17 she overlaps with her mother's account, which centres on what 'they' did to her. Here she tries to shoe-horn in a reference to the hospital's results, aligning herself to the GP and to a more doctorable narrative for the health professional (Bolden 2000). Again, in turn 25, she reformulates her mother's somewhat unspecific reference to her heart into a specific, doctorable symptom, 'not a chest pain' but a 'murmury feeling'. Although never invited, explicitly, to act as a mediator, she takes on the role of an interactional mediator. She fills in and expands information, disambiguates, makes vague accounts explicit and provides an evaluative gloss.

In Example 2, about ten minutes into the consultation, the doctor is about to take the patient's blood pressure. In the later feedback session with the researcher, he explained that by this point, he was almost certain that the patient had not had another heart attack but was presenting with symptoms brought on by stress or anxiety.

Example 2

231 D: are you under <u>stress</u> at the moment
(1.0)
232 R: she does get a bit stressed because of my dad

233 P: hearing problem
234 R: oh he just he doesn't hear very [well]
235 P: [you-] you explain to him [things]
236 R: [she] gets very- she gets frustrated with him and he- (.) it's just silly little things but she gets worked up yeah
237 D: is that getting more of a problem than it was
238 P: it's getting worse because he's- <u>he's</u> getting worse (.) deaf (.) [shouting an']
239 R: [he's getting] forgetful as well
240 P: an' course shouting at him makes him cross (.) ((to daughter)) it's the truth innit
241 R: mm
(2.0)
242 D: is it getting too much for you
(1.0)
243 P: my daughter says not to take any notice (.) but what can you-
(5.0)
((GP taking pt's blood pressure; mother and daughter exchange a glance and smile))
244 P: ((well I came here to tell the [truth innit]))
((sotto voce))
245 R: [yeah you] <u>tell</u> the truth

The doctor's social-psychological theme is met by silence from the patient, who may be co-opting her daughter to speak for her. Certainly, the daughter treats the one-second pause as a possible turn offer. She provides a context for her mother's stress while still implicating herself in this joint story of family difficulties when she categorizes the source of the difficulty as 'my dad' (turn 232). The daughter is thus presenting herself as a ratified speaker of the family story, somewhat in contrast to a typical professional interpreter's role as a ratified speaker in facilitating clearer information and negotiating more interactional space (Wadensjö 1998). Her mother's explanation of the 'hearing problem' (turn 233) is reformulated out of the more medical arena into an imaginable social scene in which the irritation of trying to communicate with an elderly hard-of-hearing person bubbles over. Again, while the mother tells the story from her perspective of how cross her husband becomes, the daughter, antiphonally, provides a perspective on her mother: 'she gets frustrated with him' (turn 236), providing an evaluative thread to the mother's story while also aligning to the doctor.

At this point, the alignment of the daughter as an interactional mediator changes as her mother draws her away from speaking *for* her to speaking *with* her and so re-frames the encounter. The mother draws her daughter into a micro conspiracy in which she reiterates her position that she came to tell the truth (turn 244). In the following turn, the daughter is emphatic in her encouragement and moves from animating her mother's words and implicit stance to actively reinforcing them. In both parts of the sequence, she is acting as a mediator, but the shift towards the end makes her an advocate, an explicit champion of her mothers' concerns.

In Example 3, which occurs about two minutes after Example 2, the doctor is trying to persuade the patient that she does not have a heart problem.

Example 3

266 D: but it's- it's not your heart
(2.0)
267 P: uh why do they tell us different things
268 D: Well [nobody's saying anything different]
269 R: [who s- who said different] thing- who said different things
270 D: [who's saying]
271 P: [the hospi-]
272 D: anything different
273 P: the hospital
(1.5)
274 D: [well]
275 R: [well] they didn't they kept you in [they did]
276 D: [they kept you-]
277 R: some tests and they sent you- [sent]
278 D: [yes]
279 R: you home
280 D: they s- they told you it wasn't your heart as well (.) cos that's what it says on the letter if they told you (.) it would have been (.) what they would have said at [this time]
281 P: [no I] mean this time when I went in the second time
282 D: yeah it wasn't your heart this time (1.0) all the heart tests are normal (0.5) that's what it says in the letter
283 P: did they sa- did that say
284 D: yes
285 P: they never said anything to me
286 D: mm (.) well (. .) do you believe me
((touches her knee))
287 P: of course I believe you
288 D: you looked a little uncertain there (.) we've just clarified that one (.) now if it's not your heart then we have to think it might be something else

As can be seen, the doctor meets with some resistance when he tells the patient she does not have a heart problem at the moment. Her lack of information, possible confusion and possible mix-up over the two different occasions when she has been in hospital with a suspected heart attack may all be summarized in her rebuttal: 'why do they tell us different things' (turn 267). Over the next few turns, the daughter aligns with the doctor in refuting her mother's claim. First, the daughter echoes the doctor and then he echoes her, both of them stating the facts in order to shift the patient's stance. In turns 280 and 282, the doctor then draws on the medical evidence and the authority of the hospital letter as persuasive devices and, at this point, the daughter takes a back seat. At this juncture she is not needed to do any institutional work; nor is she needed when the doctor, in turn 286, has a conspiratorial moment with his patient, 'do you believe me?'. In the earlier example, a similar moment between the mother and the daughter was about truth-telling (Example 2, line 240); here it is a moment about belief/trust. In both cases, the moment restores the patient's position after a momentary relegation to third party, or even merely 'overhearer' in the interaction. And, arguably, this moment of intimacy may have been influenced by the doctor overhearing this previous conspiratorial chat between the mother and the daughter.

The daughter's role in the early part of this extract is less about co-narrating and more about managing a mismatch in framing. While the doctor is in the frame of reassurance (the patient has not had a heart attack, which is good news), the mother treats it negatively as yet another example of institutions out to confuse her. While earlier in the consultation the daughter has skilfully inserted context and stance to amplify her mother's somewhat elliptical story, here she more forcefully challenges her mother three times (turns 270, 277 and 279). She seems to be taking on a gatekeeping role, aligning with the doctor to reassure her mother that she has not had another heart attack. We may conclude that 'frame work' is harder than 'narrative work', especially when, as the mediating companion, the re-framing is coupled with co-narrating (275, 277).

In Example 4, the final example from this particular consultation, we see the daughter's role change again.

Example 4

409 D: well why don't you have a think talk about it between yourselves first because you're two of the key players and see because it sounds like you're getting to a stage where it's getting a bit too much

410 R: I mean Mum- I think Mum needs to try and not worry too much I know it's easier said than done though isn't it

411 D: yes
412 R: I mean I'm the same cos I'm a worrier and I know I mean like my mum and the slightest thing
413 D: but the problem is that erm it's coming to a bit of a head

This extract, nearing the end of the consultation, shifts the role of the daughter from mediator to carer, as the doctor implicates them both in the management plan. The daughter takes the lead in responding to it, using herself as an example, 'cos I'm a worrier' (turn 412), to involve the doctor in understanding the complexity of the situation and so relegating her mother, momentarily, to third-party status. The three-way alignment that the daughter has shown, in different stages of the consultation, is summed up here. She speaks *to* the doctor, shaping the patient's problems to the institution (what has to be tackled is 'not worrying'); she speaks *for* her mother (what a high level of worrying her mother experiences); and she speaks *with* her mother (aligning her own worrying nature to her mother's).

The daughter's work is to make the implicit explicit, expanding on her mother's stance; to disambiguate and act as a mediator between the voice of medicine and the patient's lifeworld narrative voice (Mishler 1984); and in doing so to take on an advocacy role. Often this means that she offers an explanation or clarification unasked – interactional work which would otherwise have been done by the doctor. She co-narrates with her mother but also with the doctor. However, she goes much further than this conventional role in her interactional mediation and advocacy as she expands her mother's stance, commenting on her mother's perspective as well. And threaded through all this is the intimacy of their shared history and lives which only a relative or close partner or friend could bring to the consultation.

Much of the literature on triadic consultations is critical of this advocate and interventionist role. The majority of critiques concern the role of the designated interpreter, but there are also critiques of triadic consultations more generally (Beisecker 1989; Vickers *et al.* 2015). Beisecker labels the third party as 'watchdog', 'significant other' or 'surrogate patient' – all used as rather negative terms – and concludes, as do Vickers and co-authors, that it is a matter of control. While the third party appears supportive, the patient's voice is suppressed and the relationship between doctor and patient muted. However, we have tried to show that it is not a matter of *appearing* supportive only, but of using the trust and intimacy between the mother and the daughter to produce a jointly constructed co-operative plan where the patient may sometimes be the overhearer, but can benefit from being in this role. Speaking *for* someone is not a simple matter of depriving them of their voice. Indeed, the patient's voice may be amplified by the family member most concerned for their wellbeing – as appears to be the case here.

The interpreter-mediated consultation

This consultation is with a middle-aged Turkish woman and her daughter, probably in her early 20s, who acts as the lay interpreter. The doctor is a nationally recognized general practitioner. She also specializes in mental health issues. The following data extracts are taken from the same consultation. The Turkish expressions are marked in bold and the translated expressions are in italic. Example 5 begins after greetings and the doctor first addresses the daughter and turns to the mother.

Example 5

07 D: how can I help your mum
08 R: **agrin nedir** *(what is your pains)*
09 P: **karnim agriyor sirtim agriyor bacagim agriyor** ( ) *(I have got stomach ache pain in my back and in my leg)*
10 R: she say she's got pains in her chest and on her back and then it's a different pain in her knee ( ) up there
11 D: okay does she want to tell me about the pain in her chest a little bit
12 R: **nasil bir karin agrisi** *(what kind of pain do you have)*
13 P: **karnim buradan agriyor birde karnimin ortasindan agriyor beraber tam ortasindan** ( ) *(I have pain here in my stomach then just in the middle of my stomach and together ( ) in the middle)*
14 R: so it starts here and goes to the back of her back so it's like the pain is from there to the back of her back ((daughter indicates the location of the pain))

The mother, who does not speak English at all, has come to the clinic complaining about her painful stomach, back and knees. In addition to translating her mother's words, the daughter clarifies the symptoms, adding a layer of precision to the patient's story ('it's a different pain in her knee', turn 11; 'up there', turn 12; and 'so it starts here and goes to the back', turn 18). This filling in and expanding of information pre-empts possible follow-up questions by the doctor and is similar to the role taken on by Mrs S's daughter in the mediated consultation in English in making the story more doctorable. In both cases, the daughters as carers draw on their 'insider knowledge' of the patient's situation to assist the doctor in reaching a workable diagnosis. They both seem to be acting as gatekeepers but also as amplifiers of the patient's voice, drawing the patient's world into the gaze of the doctor.

After the history taking, in Example 6 the doctor turns to the daughter to ask about psychosocial symptoms.

Example 6

61 D: your mother doesn't drink or smoke =does she=
62 R: =no=
63 D: ((laughs)) unlike the next =generation presumably=
64 R: =((laughs))=
65 D: ((laughs)) where are you from from Turkey
66 R: yeah
67 D: your mother seems a bit down is this how she normally is
68 R: no she is just suffering cos just her knee is really hurting her
69 D: right cos she seems quite sad and quite
70 R: ((laughs))
71 P: **ne oluyor** *(what is happening)*
72 R: **pek mutlu degilsin diyor** *(she said you don't seem very happy)*
73 P: **mutluyum canim** *(I am happy my dear)*
74 D: her knee is hurting knee's been hurting her for a long time hasn't it
75 R: yeah
76 P: **dizimin agrisi cok fazla** *(I have got very strong pain in my knee)*
77 R: because they usually it's because of the weight but it's just
78 P: ( )
((sounds of clothes shuffling))

At the start of this extract, and in contrast to Example 5, the doctor has co-opted the daughter into the interaction, ratifying her contribution not as a lay interpreter but as a full conversational partner when she comments about the strong possibility that the younger generation may smoke and drink. She then, at turn 67, introduces the theme of the patient's general wellbeing. As in the earlier case study discussed above (see Example 2), it is when psychosocial topics are introduced that the doctor talks directly to the interpreter or mediator. But, as with the earlier case, the patient intervenes in turn 71 so that she is not sidelined by the doctor–daughter discussion. This intervention seems to confirm the daughter's explanation that her mother is not sad but in pain. However, unlike with Mrs S, whose comments are all hearable by the doctor, this remark 'I am happy dear' (turn 73) is not translated. At this point the formal (and seen as ideal) turn-taking system in professional interpreter mediated consultations, in which each turn by patient and interpreter must be interpreted (Li 2015), is not present.[1] However, the daughter's absence of a translation but insistence that the knee is hurting may imply that sadness is not the problem, as shown in Example 7.

Example 7

79 D: she's keeping warm with (your long johns)
((D touches patient's knee))
80 R: ((laughs))
81 D: ((laughs))
82 P: **agriyor usumesin diye iste** *(it is painful I wear those to protect myself from cold)*
83 D: where =does it hurt=
84 R: (she only) put one layer on today ((laughs))

As with Mrs S's encounter, above, the doctor shifts from third to second person and back again quite routinely. In turn 79, the doctor switches from 'she' to 'your' in mid-utterance and reinforces this shift in attention with her bodily conduct by touching the patient's knee. The patient responds in Turkish, showing her moral self to the doctor (turn 82), as someone who is sensible in looking after herself. The daughter does not translate this but aligns with the doctor, maintaining the theme ('she only put one layer on today', turn 84), sharing the humour of long johns with her. But, arguably, she is also defending her mother with this utterance, possibly indicating that her mother's one layer is to ease any physical examination or that her mother is sensible but not over-protective of herself. While a conventional analysis might simply critique the daughter's conduct, we can read it in a more sympathetic light. It indexes her janus-like role in representing her mother and also sharing the humorous aspect of the underwear with the doctor, underscoring the importance of maintaining friendly relations with the doctor.

As well as moments when lifeworld and moral themes are not translated, there are also misalignments when different functions of the doctor's utterances are filtered out from the daughter's translation for her mother. For example, in Example 8 below, the doctor's diagnosis of the patient's knee is not translated.

Example 8

103 D: the other thing is she's got quite bad knee there when you feel it you feel it scrape has your mother had any x-rayed
104 R: erm **x-ray olmustu senin dizinde degil mi** *(you have had any x-ray)*
105 P: **belimden mi dizim mi dizimden olmustu** *(from my back or knee I have had from my knee)*
106 R: **x-ray olduydu** *(you have had x-ray)*
107 R: yeah she's had an x-ray on her

The misalignment here is that while the doctor wants to convey her hands-on diagnosis as well as discuss X–rays, the daughter orientates to the more factual aspects of the diagnosis. It is plausible that the daughter wants to protect her mother from this negative diagnosis, choosing protection over autonomy, or, as elsewhere, editing out those aspects which she may perceive as not strictly pertinent to driving the management plan forward. Or it may be a matter of competence – she may not be able to make sense of or retain or translate the idea of the knee 'scraping.'

Given the potential for misalignments in multiparty talk in this kind of clinical setting, great communicative dexterity is required on the part of the doctor. In the final data example below (Example 9) we see how the doctor, while trying to attain the primary goal of the consultation, i.e. the discussion of treatment options, orients to the daughter (who we must remember is a third party in this encounter) as well as the patient, even to the extent of allowing the daughter as lay interpreter a momentary role as second patient in the room.

Prior to turn 120, the doctor has just told the daughter that her mother's knee is quite bad and that she is to be referred to a specialist. The daughter becomes quite tearful at this point. So, sadness is an issue in this encounter.

Example 9

120 D: What's the matter
121 R: I don't know ((tearful))
122 D: What's the matter I'm gonna have to ask your mother now in Turkish why you're upset
123 R: ((sobbing))
124 P: **ne oldu** *(what happened)*
125 D: ((to patient)) why is she upset
126 P: (   )
127 D: ((to daughter)) why are you upset
128 R: I don't know I get ((tearful voice)) I don't like to see my mum upset like that (   ) her knee is really (   ) can't (   ) some place (   )=

129 D: =I know I'm sure she's in a lot of pain actually which is why I'm going to refer her to a specialist but is that why you're so upset
130 R: uhm
131 D: so both of you are looking sad I was right
132 P: **ne oldu kotu bir sey mi dedi** *(what happened did she say something bad)*
133 R: **yo** *(no)* ((tearful))
134 D: you've got other brothers and sisters
135 R: hmm two brothers and two sisters
136 D: are you the youngest
137 R: hmm
138 D: ((to patient)) the baby your daughter is the baby the youngest
139 P: **ne diyor** *(what she said)*
140 R: **bir sey yok** *(nothing)*
141 D: alright

As the daughter becomes increasingly tearful, the doctor's gaze turns to her. The interpreter becomes, for a moment, the patient and is addressed directly as such. With an uncomprehending legitimate patient and a tearful interpreter-patient, the doctor has a complicated emotional and moral landscape to deal with. She uses several strategies. Firstly, she tries to clarify the reasons why the daughter is upset (turn 120), then twice aligns with the mother, first to ask about, and then to comment on, the daughter (turns 122 and 125). This need to align sympathetically with the mother while her daughter seems the most needy of the two overrides the obvious language barrier between the mother and the doctor. Again, the daughter does not translate the doctor's attempts to seek ways of supporting the tearful young woman, but seems to treat the information about her family as a side-sequence. The doctor's 'alright' (turn 141) closes this moment and the mother and the daughter return to their conventional roles, with no clear resolution for the mother about whether the doctor has 'said something bad' (turn 132).

7.5 Discussion: The role of the mediator/interpreter – a tripartite continuum

There are clearly differences in these two triadic consultations. However, a comparison suggests that the bilingual one where the daughter acts as interpreter and the monolingual one where the daughter is the companion have more in common than the literature on interpreting versus other triadic encounters implies. There is clearly some information loss in the lay interpreter-mediated consultation, which is not so evident in the monolingual encounter. However, in the latter case, the daughter frequently latches onto her mother's utterances or takes the unfilled pauses, thus possibly subduing her mother's voice and her agendas. There is also a difference in the age and status of the two third parties. Mrs S's daughter is middle-aged and displays confidence and experience in helping her mother. Mrs T's daughter is young and appears relatively inexperienced as a carer. She plays a much greater role in explicating her mother's stance and in evaluating her situation at home. These differences may contribute to some of the differences in the two encounters.

Nevertheless, what is striking about these two encounters are the main similarities in role and interactional alignments. Both daughters act as mediators, particularly in the early stages of the consultation involving symptom presentation and history taking, and in the diagnostic phase. The conventional sequential structuring of doctor to interpreter to patient to interpreter to doctor (Li 2015) makes this obvious in the second case study, especially during the symptoms presentation and history-taking phases (turns 7–77, not shown in the examples). But even in the first case, there are examples of the daughter clarifying, disambiguating and making information more expectable. Both daughters also fill in and extend their mothers' formulations and so both do co-narrating work, although as mentioned above, Mrs S's daughter does more of the evaluating stage of the narrative than the younger woman does in Mrs T's case. We could argue that both do linguistic work and both do gatekeeping and advocacy and are involved in the interactional management of doctor–patient relations and their own relations with both of the other two parties.

The daughter as companion, the daughter as lay interpreter and the two doctors, on occasions, give third-party status to the patients. Again this can be seen in the sequential structuring at different moments, marked by third-person referencing and tag questions. It is also evident in the shift to third person and in the ways in which psychosocial topics are maintained and developed between third parties and doctors (for example the brief discussion on whether young Turkish people smoke and drink). This sharing of themes between the doctors and the two daughters is one of the skilful ways in which both sides manage the complex and potentially face-threatening aspects of the triadic encounter, when any of the three can potentially become the third party. In both case studies, the shift to a psychosocial topic produces third-party status for the two patients but both intervene to re-enter the interaction by commenting on their situation.

Both the lay interpreter and the companion align to the institutional aspects of the encounter, but in rather different ways. Mrs S's daughter uses her mediation role to make her mother's presentation of self, symptoms and wider context more doctorable. For example, she translates her mother's rather vague description about her heart into a specific metaphor, 'murmury feeling'. Mrs T's daughter also works to make her mother's talk more doctorable but tends to align to the institution in a more gatekeeping way (Davidson 2000) by treating the lifeworld aspects as side sequences that do not need valorizing through translation.

Both daughters are carers, as well as having a mediating role. Their presence in the consulting room establishes this, but it is also clear in the remarkable intimate, emotional and off-stage work they both do in disclosing their feelings and anxieties about their mothers. Mrs S confides, *sotto voce*, to her daughter that they had agreed that she would tell the truth and in the final stages of the consultation, the daughter discloses her own worried self in commenting on her mother's home situation. The young daughter's emotional labour as a carer is expressed more directly when she bursts into tears and her role as interpreter is temporarily suspended. In all these instances the supportive, collaborative and intimate relations between mother and daughter suggest a level of trust unlikely to be found in consultations with professional interpreters (although for a counter example see Wadensjö, this issue, where the professional interpreter seems to build trust between patient and doctor). Both examples are notable for the display of feelings and the close and loving relationships between mother and daughter, punctuated by moments of frustration, and the caring respect tempered by glimpses of humour shown by each doctor to both patients and the daughters who accompany them.

Finally, all three parties attend to the complex participation frameworks in which three people manoeuvre around what is traditionally a two-way interaction. All three find intimate moments, local confederations, with one another when the main track of the consultation is subverted. This is done through *sotto voce* talk, talk in a language incomprehensible to the other which yet draws them in and in non-verbal moments of touch to counterpoint other moments when the patient has been constructed as a third party.

Professional interpreter (gatekeeper)	*Professional interpreter* (impartial)	*Cultural mediator* (advocate)	*Lay/family* interpreter	*Companion* mediator	*Chauffeur*

Figure 7.1 The role continuum.

Interpreter as social and linguistic intermediary

While the healthcare literature has been largely concerned with issues of provision and accuracy, the sociolinguistic literature has focused on the social and interactional aspects of the mediated encounter. The latter studies present the interpreter as a full participant, with social agency and interactional rights and not a mere conduit (Ebden *et al.* 1988). In much of this literature, where the interpreter sits in relation to the continuum (see Figure 7.1) is less important than how the conversational flow is framed and managed (Wadenjö 1998; Roy 1999; Coupland and Coupland 2000; Li *et al.* 2017). Sociolinguistic analysis has also examined how professional interpreters employed by an institution, such as a hospital, can act as gatekeepers. They manage the interaction, actively evaluating the patient's discourse to save the doctor's, and therefore the institution's, time (Davidson 2000).

The social and interactional lens transforms the mediated consultation into a complex negotiation of talk and social relations and provides analytic frameworks that allow interesting insights into the various roles called up in mediated encounters, from institutional gatekeeping to the intimate advocacy of a family member, as discussed here. Unlike previous studies, we have looked beyond the mechanisms of interaction to how trust, confidence and feelings are threaded through the family mediating and interpreting work.

The data analytical findings lead us to propose a role continuum to capture the dynamics of mediation, as in Figure 7.1. Although these might appear as discreet roles, with professional/paid interpreters on the left and family interpreters and mediators on the right, there are elements of all of these interactional roles in the data discussed above. There is evidence of gatekeeping and more impartial interpretation and re-wording, of elaboration and expansion to make the patient's utterances more doctorable, of advocacy, of mediation of the more emotional and intimate aspects of the mother/daughter relationships and of some 'chauffeuring' work, driving the consultation towards the daughters' goals.

7.6 Conclusion

In this paper we have explored the dynamics of triadic interaction in the primary care setting, where the co-present third party positions herself either as a companion or as a mediator, the latter being the case when the patient has a low level of proficiency in the language of the clinic. Our findings show that such positioning cannot be simplistically framed in either/or terms, as shifts in interactional footing are routinely identifiable.

Family interpreters and mediators are also carers, and have three different footings which continuously re-frame the triadic consultation. They speak *for* patients, in a representative role as ambassadors. They speak *with* the patients, as advocates of the patients' view and often echoing their stances and emotions. They also speak *to* the doctor, both directly and when the doctor is an overhearer. They mediate between the relative and the institution in making the patient's story more doctorable, summarizing or eliminating aspects of the talk which they do not see as salient for the doctor, in a gatekeeping role. But this role is also subverted when they implicate themselves personally in the patient's world, living the patient's worries as in the first case study, or weeping for their mother, as in the second case study.

In many respects the lay or family interpreter has more in common with the companion in a monolingual setting than with the professional interpreter. Both family interpreters and companions take on partisan roles, becoming spokespeople or even 'authors' in their own right, or indeed in the suppression of information, in order to accomplish tasks that they deem to be necessary, orientating to both doctor and patient. In so doing they mediate not only the interaction but also the consultation process and the feelings it elicits, and by implication the outcome of a consultation.

Most of the interpreting research literature only attends to the differences between professional and lay interpreters to air the problems with the latter and the need to replace them with professionals. It rarely looks at some of the valuable work done by lay interpreters and does not consider the triadic consultations where carers become mediators and take on linguistic and advocacy work. This study has outlined some of the commonalities between family members as monolingual carers and as lay interpreters in multilingual encounters. The social and interactional work of the companion-mediators in representing and advocating on behalf of a relative is not questioned. But a similar task undertaken by lay or family interpreters is often criticized for not being sufficiently impartial and for depriving the patient of their voice and of control in the consultation (Beisecker 1989; Vickers *et al.* 2015).

Although information loss, inaccuracies and an undermining of patient control remain potential problems in family interpreting, the value of family interpreter's understanding and commitment to the patient, who is also their relative, may bring advantages which are not widely voiced, in particular to the opportunities in such encounters for feelings to be surfaced and attended to. Some patients seem to prefer a family interpreter to a professional one and more research comparing the two will help to establish whether they are justified in their preference. Similarly, more research on the role of the carer as an active mediator will help to bring this kind of triadic consultation into focus so that its significance in producing the best outcomes for patients can also be considered.

Appendix: Transcription conventions

The following transcription conventions are adapted from Psathas (1995).

[	Overlap e.g.: T: I used to smoke [a lot B: he th]inks he's real tough
=	Latching i.e. where the next speakers turn follows on without any pause e.g.: A: I used to smoke a lot= B: = =He thinks he's real tough
(.)	Untimed brief pauses
(1)	Timed pauses in seconds
(s'pose so)	Unclear talk / possible hearings indicated by stretch of talk in parentheses
( )	Unrecognisable talk, empty brackets
((bell sounds))	Description of conversational scene
((whispered))	Description of characterizations of talk

Acknowledgments

This paper derives from the project titled Patients with Limited English and Doctors in General Practice (PLEDGE), which was funded by Sir

Siegmund Warburg's Voluntary Settlement (2001–2003). We are grateful to Marie-Jet Bekkers for her assistance during the drafting of this manuscript. We also would like to acknowledge Cecilia Wadensjö for her perceptive comments on an earlier draft of the paper.

Note

1 Out of the total of 177 turns in this three-party consultation, the doctor takes 68 turns, the daughter takes 80 turns and the patient takes only 29 turns.

References

Angelelli, Claudia V. (2005) *Medical Interpreting and Cross-Cultural Communication.* Cambridge: Cambridge University Press. https://doi.org/10.1017/CBO9780511486616

Bamberg, Michael and Alexandra Georgakopoulou (2008) Small stories as a new perspective in narrative and identity analysis. *Text & Talk* 28 (3): 377–396. https://doi.org/10.1515/TEXT.2008.018

Baraldi, Claudio and Laura Gavioli (eds) (2012) *Coordinating Participation in Dialogue Interpreting.* Amsterdam: John Benjamins. https://doi.org/10.1075/btl.102

Beisecker, Analee E. (1989) The influence of a companion on the doctor-elderly patient interaction. *Health and Communication* 1 (1): 55–70. https://doi.org/10.1207/s15327027hc0101_7

Bolden, Galina B. (2000) Toward understanding practices of medical interpreting: Interpreters' involvement in history taking. *Discourse Studies* 2 (4): 387–419. https://doi.org/10.1177/1461445600002004001

Cohen, Suzanne, Jo Moran-Ellis and Chris Smaje (1999) Children as informal interpreters in GP consultations: Pragmatics and ideology. *Sociology of Health & Illness* 21 (2): 163–186. https://doi.org/10.1111/1467-9566.00148

Cordella, Marisa (2011) A triangle that may work well: Looking through the angles of a three-way exchange in cancer medical encounters. *Discourse and Communication* 5 (4): 337–353. https://doi.org/10.1177/1750481311418100

Corsellis, Ann (2008) *Public Service Interpreting: The First Steps.* Basingstoke, UK: Palgrave Macmillan. https://doi.org/10.1057/9780230581951

Coupland, Nikolas and Justine Coupland (2000) Relational frames and pronominal address/reference: The discourse of geriatric medical triads.

In Srikant Sarangi and Malcolm Coulthard (eds) *Discourse and Social Life*, 207–229. Harlow, UK: Pearson.

Davidson, Brad (2000) The interpreter as institutional gatekeeper: The socio-linguistic role of interpreters in Spanish-English medical discourse. *Journal of Sociolinguistics* 4 (3): 379–405. https://doi.org/10.1111/1467-9481.00121

Ebden, Philip, Arvind Bhatt, Oliver J. Carey and Brian Harrison (1988) The bilingual consultation. *Lancet* (8581): 347. https://doi.org/10.1016/S0140-6736(88)91133-6

Goffman, Erving (1974) *Frame Analysis: An Essay on the Organization of Experience*. New York: Harper & Row.

Goffman, Erving (1981) *Forms of Talk*. Oxford: Blackwell.

Goffman, Erving (1983) The interaction order. *American Sociological Review* 48 (1): 1–17. https://doi.org/10.2307/2095141

Green, Judith, Caroline Free, Vanita Bhavnani and Tony Newman (2005) Translators and mediators: Bilingual young people's accounts of their interpreting work in health care. *Social Science and Medicine* 60 (9): 2097–2110. https://doi.org/10.1016/j.socscimed.2004.08.067

Greenhalgh, Trisha, Nadia Robb and Graham Scambler (2006) Communicative and strategic action in interpreted consultations in primary healthcare: A Habermassian perspective. *Social Science & Medicine* 63 (5): 1170–1187. https://doi.org/10.1016/j.socscimed.2006.03.033

Haffner, Larry (1992) Translation is not enough: Interpreting in a medical setting. *Western Journal of Medicine* 157 (3): 255–259.

Hale, Sandra B. (2004) *The Discourse of Course Interpreting: Discourse Practices of the Law, the Witness and the Interpreter*. Amsterdam: John Benjamins. https://doi.org/10.1075/btl.52

Labov, William and Joshua Waletzky (1967) Narrative analysis: Oral versions of personal experience. In June Helm (ed.) *Essays on the Verbal and Visual Arts*, 12–44. Seattle: University of Washington Press.

Li, Shuangyu (2015) Nine types of turn-taking in interpreter-mediated GP consultations. *Applied Linguistics Review* 6 (1): 73–96. https://doi.org/10.1515/applirev-2015-0004

Li, Shuangyu, Jennifer Gerwing, Demi Krystallidou, Angela Rowlands, Antoon Cox and Peter Pype (2017) Interaction – A missing piece of the jigsaw in interpreter-mediated medical consultation models. *Patient Education and Counseling* 100 (9): 1769–1771. https://doi.org/10.1016/j.pec.2017.04.021

Meyer, Bernd (2012). *Ad hoc* interpreting for partially language-proficient patients: Participation in multilingual constellations. In Claudio Baraldi and Laura Gavioli (eds) *Coordinating Participation in Dialogue*

Interpreting, 99–113. Amsterdam: John Benjamins. https://doi.org/10.1075/btl.102.05mey

Mishler, Elliot G. (1984) *The Discourse of Medicine: Dialectics of Medical Interviews*. Norwood, NJ: Ablex.

Moss, Becky and Celia Roberts (2005) Explanations, explanations, explanations: How do patients with limited English construct narrative accounts in multi-lingual, multi-ethnic settings, and how can GPs interpret them? *Family Practice* 22 (4): 412–418. https://doi.org/10.1093/fampra/cmi037

Pöchhacker, Franz (2004) *Introducing Interpreting Studies*. London: Routledge. https://doi.org/10.4324/9780203504802

Psathas, George (1995) 'Talk and social structure' and 'studies of work'. *Human Studies* 18 (2–3): 139–155. https://doi.org/10.1007/BF01323207

Putsch, Robert W. III (1985) Cross-cultural communication: The special case of interpreters in health care. *Journal of the American Medical Association* 254 (23): 3344–3348. https://doi.org/10.1001/jama.1985.03360230076027

Raymond, Chase W. (2014a) Conveying information in the interpreter-mediated medical visit: The case of epistemic brokering. *Patient Education and Counseling* 97 (1): 38–46. https://doi.org/10.1016/j.pec.2014.05.020

Raymond, Chase W. (2014b) Epistemic brokering in the interpreter-mediated medical visit: Negotiating 'patient's side' and 'doctor's side' knowledge. *Research on Language and Social Interaction* 47 (4): 426–446. https://doi.org/10.1080/08351813.2015.958281

Robb, Nadia and Trisha Greenhalgh (2006) 'You have to cover up the words of the doctor': The mediation of trust in interpreted consultations in primary healthcare. *Journal of Healthcare Organisation and Management* 20 (5): 434–455. https://doi.org/10.1108/14777260610701803

Roberts, Celia, Srikant Sarangi and Becky Moss (2004) 'Presentation of self and symptom in primary care consultations involving patients from non-English speaking backgrounds. *Communication & Medicine* 1 (2): 159–169. https://doi.org/10.1515/come.2004.1.2.159

Roy, Cynthia B. (1999) *Interpreting as a Discourse Process*. New York: Oxford University Press.

Sarangi, Srikant (2012) The intercultural complex in healthcare encounters: A discourse analytical perspective. In Nivritti G. Patil and Cindy L. K. Lam (eds) *Making Sense in Communication*, 13–24. Hong Kong: Institute of Medical and Health Sciences Education.

Schouten, Barbara C. and Ludwien Meeuwesen (2006) Cultural differences in medical communication: A review of the literature. *Patient Education & Counselling* 64 (1–3): 21–34. https://doi.org/10.1016/j.pec.2005.11.014

Silverman, David (1987) *Communication and Medical Practice: Social Relations in the Clinic*. London: Sage.

Singy, Pascal and Patrice Guex (2005) The interpreter's role with immigrant patients: Contrasted points of view. *Communication & Medicine* 2 (1): 45–51. https://doi.org/10.1515/come.2005.2.1.45

Stokes, Randall and John P. Hewitt (1976) Aligning actions. *American Sociological Review* 41 (5): 838–849. https://doi.org/10.2307/2094730

Swinglehurst, Deborah, Celia Roberts, Shuangyu Li, Orest Weber and Pascal Singy (2014) Beyond the 'dyad': A qualitative re-evaluation of the changing clinical consultation. *BMJ Open* 4 (9): e006017. https://doi.org/10.1136/bmjopen-2014-006017

Tannen, Deborah and Cynthia Wallat (1983) Doctor/mother/child communication: Linguistic analysis of a paediatric interaction. In Alexandra D. Todd and Sue Fisher (eds) *The Social Organisation of Doctor-Patient Communication*, 203–219. Washington, DC: Center for Applied Linguistics.

Tsai, Mei-hui (2007) Who gets to talk?: An interactive framework evaluating companion effects in geriatric triads. *Communication & Medicine* 4 (1): 37–49. https://doi.org/10.1515/CAM.2007.005

Vertovec, Steven (2007) Super-diversity and its implications. *Ethnic and Racial Studies* 30 (6): 1024–1054. https://doi.org/10.1080/01419870701599465

Vertovec, Steven (2010) Towards post-multilingualism? Changing communities, conditions and contexts of diversity. *International Science Journal* 199: 83–95. https://doi.org/10.1111/j.1468-2451.2010.01749.x

Vickers, Caroline H., Ryan Goble and Sharon K. Deckert (2015) Third party interaction in the medical context: Code-switching and control. *Journal of Pragmatics* 84: 154–171. https://doi.org/10.1016/j.pragma.2015.05.009

Wadensjö, Cecilia (1998) *Interpreting as Interaction*. Harlow, UK: Addison Wesley Longman.

Celia Roberts is Professor Emerita in Sociolinguistics and Applied Linguistics, King's College London. Her publications in language and inequality in institutional contexts include *Language and Discrimination* (with Davies and Jupp; Longman, 1992), *Achieving Understanding* (with Bremer *et al.*; Longman, 1996), *Talk, Work and Institutional Order* (with Sarangi; De Gruyter, 1996) *Language Learners as Ethnographers* (with Byram *et al.*; Multilingual Matters, 2001); *Performance Features in Clinical Skills Assessment* (with Atkins and Hawthorne; King's College London, 2014); and *Linguistic Penalties and the Job Interview* (Equinox, 2021), which was shortlisted for the BAAL book prize in 2022 and examines the inequalities migrants face in job interviewing.

Address for correspondence: Faculty of Social Science and Public Policy, King's College London, Strand, London WC2R 2LS, UK.

Srikant Sarangi was Professor in Humanities and Medicine and Director of the Danish Institute of Humanities and Medicine (DIHM) between 2013 and 2021 at Aalborg University, Denmark, where he continues as Adjunct Professor. Between 1993 and 2013, he was Professor in Language and Communication and Director of the Health Communication Research Centre at Cardiff University, UK, where he continues as Emeritus Professor. In recent years he has been Visiting Professor in many countries, including Finland, Hong Kong, Malaysia, Norway and Qatar. He is author and editor of twelve books, guest editor of ten journal special issues and has published more than 250 journal articles and book chapters in leading journals. Since 1998 he is the editor of *TEXT & TALK: An Interdisciplinary Journal of Language, Discourse and Communication Studies* (formerly *TEXT*) as well as the founding editor, since 2004, of both *Communication & Medicine* and *Journal of Applied Linguistics and Professional Practice* (formerly *Journal of Applied Linguistics*). He is also general editor of the book series *Studies in Communication in Organisations and Professions* (*SCOPE*). Address for correspondence: Department of Communication and Psychology, Aalborg University, Rendsburggade 14, 9000 Aalborg, Denmark. Email: sarangi@ikp.aau.dk

8 The comparison of shared decision making in monolingual and bilingual health encounters

Charlene Pope & Jason Roberson

8.1 Introduction: Significance of language-linked health disparities

According to the US Agency for Healthcare Research and Quality (2017), health disparities reports from 2012 to 2015 showed that some gaps are narrowing, but Hispanics in the US continue to receive worse access to and quality of care than non-Hispanics. Hispanic patients whose primary language is Spanish experience particular barriers in accessing and using health services (Smith 2010) and report poorer health than primary English speakers (Sentell and Braun 2012). This gap persists despite US policy mandates that have increased availability of medical interpreters (US Department of Health and Human Services 2003, 2013; Chen *et al.* 2007). How provider–patient communication and decision making differ between monolingual encounters and bilingual limited English proficiency (LEP) encounters when interpreters are present constitutes an emerging area of concern (Carter-Pokras *et al.* 2004; Van Cleave *et al.* 2014). This paper focuses on shared decision making, defined as the active involvement and participation of physician and patient during a medical encounter, in which they are both involved in setting the agenda and sharing information, considering the patient's preferences, negotiating a consensus for the preferred treatment, and reaching an agreement about the treatment plan (Elwyn *et al.* 2016).

Ethnicity and language contribute to disparities in health services (Fiscella *et al.* 2002; Haviland *et al.* 2012), though the specific communication practices associated with the production of disparities remain to be identified (Schwei *et al.* 2016). Previous analysis demonstrates that communication contributes to differing perceptions in the quality of care (Palmer *et al.* 2014), and more than their monolingual counterparts, patients with LEP report dissatisfaction with care and difficulties using health services (Weech-Maldonado *et al.* 2008; Balakrishnan *et al.* 2016). The presence of trained interpreters may reduce some disparities (Karliner *et al.* 2007; Lindholm *et al.* 2012), but even when interpreters are present, Hispanic patients report less information, less satisfaction, and exhibit decreased subsequent compliance (Menendez *et al.* 2015). Additionally, one of the largest studies of language discordance and interpreter use (Ngo-Metzger *et al.* 2007) found Hispanic patients with LEP also tend to rate the interpersonal care they receive as lower in quality. Even with interpreter use, patients with LEP in a study of diabetes had poorer outcomes than the monolingual patients (Njeru *et al.* 2017), which suggests the impact of LEP on medical outcomes.

Similar disparities have been observed in studies regarding the role of medical interpreters in other countries and in multiple languages. In a study of 16 consultations in Canada (Leanza *et al.* 2010), trained interpreters tended to follow a 'neutral message' approach that aligned with the physicians' biomedical agenda, and which often excluded the patient's unspoken concerns, emotions, sources of resistance and personal contexts, otherwise known as the lifeworld (Mishler 1984). By contrast, studies of LEP consultations in Australia have found that physicians often underuse trained interpreters, and speak less with patients who are LEP and have interpreters when compared with consultations with English-speaking patients. These LEP patients receive less information about their condition, and tend to have their high-intensity cues ignored (Butow *et al.* 2011; Phillips and Travaglia 2011; Blay *et al.* 2018). Similarly, a study from the UK found that when 12 visits of patients with LEP and interpreters were compared with English-only patients who had diabetes, LEP patients said less, asked fewer questions, received less humor and discussion about their feelings or personal contexts, and had interpreters who sometimes changed the meaning of statements or omitted what was said (Seale *et al.* 2013). These patterns imply that shared decision making may also differ, as found in a US-based study of cancer counseling (Kamara *et al.* 2018) in which patients with LEP had little participation in medical decision making. More generally, Hispanics, whether primarily English- or Spanish-speaking, receive less patient-centered care and psychosocial talk (Beach *et al.* 2010).

This study builds on recommendations that decision making and communication require more study in ethnically and linguistically diverse populations (Wilson-Stronks *et al.* 2008). The purpose of this study is to systematically compare real-time communication of health service interactions in bilingual prenatal visits with a professional interpreter present with monolingual encounters with similar prenatal agendas, looking for variations in shared decision making. With roots in Title VI of the Civil Rights Act (Chen *et al.* 2007), Section 1557 of the Patient Protection and Affordable Care Act 2016, entitled *Ensuring Meaningful Access for Individuals with Limited English Proficiency*, requires that persons with LEP be offered trained medical interpreters who have gone through a qualification process that varies by facility (US Department of Health and Human Services 2016), but does not require interpreters be certified, though a national certification process is available (National Board of Certification for Medical Interpreters 2016a, 2016b). Interpreters in this study had received formal training and qualification required by the involved hospital and this assignment was their only role in the hospital.

8.2 Communication and shared decision making with LEP

Hispanics who report dissatisfaction with their care also report less reassurance and support from their physicians and lower quality of care (Morales *et al.* 2000; Brooks *et al.* 2016). Further, Hispanic patients who are LEP and use interpreters are more likely to have their responses ignored (Rivadeneyra *et al.* 2000) and are less likely to receive rapport building (Aranguri *et al.* 2006) than English-speaking patients as components of shared decision making. Satisfaction (Little *et al.* 2001; October 2016), adherence (Beach *et al.* 2005; Kuntz *et al.* 2014), and health status (Franks *et al.* 2005; Plewnia *et al.* 2016) have been associated with patient participation and shared decision making, though primarily in monolingual encounters. As a beginning to explaining bilingual variations, Roberts *et al.* (2005) demonstrate differences in opening sequences of health encounters for patients who do not speak the societal language. In an exploratory study of interactions between physicians and immigrant patients in the Netherlands (Suurmond and Seeleman 2006), self-report in interviews suggested barriers to shared decision making decreased dialogue and information exchange, though the interactions themselves were not examined. However, though review of studies with persons who are LEP has found that the use of professional interpreters *may* decrease errors and improve understanding, use of services, satisfaction with care, and clinical outcomes (Karliner *et al.* 2007), the effect of bilingual communication in health encounters with on-site professional interpreters may vary as regards shared decision making, process, and outcomes (Hsieh 2006; Van Cleave 2014), and this interaction requires closer investigation.

As a type of speech event with a formalized ritual structure that restricts options for participants (Saville-Troike 2003), the prenatal visit may limit opportunities for shared decision making when compared to other types of care (Tucker Edmonds 2014), particularly for those with lower socioeconomic status. In a Scottish study of pregnant women (Docherty *et al.* 2012), a comparison of those identified as most and least deprived showed that those most socioeconomically deprived women felt the least connected to their care, described less effective communication, and indicated least opportunity for shared decision making.

Although shared decision making is advocated for prenatal care (Kirkham *et al.* 2005; Nieuwenhuijze *et al.* 2014), few studies have examined the process of shared decision making in this type of encounter for monolingual women and their physicians. In a review of 155 studies of decision aids used in shared decision making (Tucker Edmonds 2014), only 29% involved reproductive health decisions and none addressed the process of shared decision making in the process of prenatal visits, despite advocating it as a promising approach for obstetricians/gynecologists and the women they serve. Similarly, although an expert international panel of providers, policy makers, educators, researchers, and care users has defined a set of quality criteria and professional competencies related to shared decision making in prenatal care (Nieuwenhuijze *et al.* 2014), the components of shared decision making in the interaction of prenatal visits are less described. We were unable to identify studies of shared decision making in recorded prenatal visits with Hispanic women, other than interviews of perceived patient-centeredness queried through *post hoc* recall (Tandon *et al.* 2005).

As a discourse process, a prenatal visit between a patient with LEP, their physician and a qualified medical interpreter may differ from a monolingual encounter in a variety of ways. Medical interpreters are taught to echo the second-language speaker by using the first person and not to intrude, but their position as a third speech partner in the medical encounter affects the usual sequences of turn-taking in conversation and they must make constant decisions and adjustments based on both linguistic and cultural meanings (Jiang *et al.* 2014). The sequences of conversational turns may involve greetings and expected responses, questions and answers, complaints and denials, raising of topics or the offering of explanations (Schegloff 2007). In medical communication, cultural differences may influence explanatory models of health and illness, values, preferences in provider–patient relationships, and social biases or prejudices (Schouten and Meeuwesen 2006; Flynn *et al.* 2014). Despite this cultural influence, the traditional interpreter role requires that the interpreter remain neutral, interpret everything that is said accurately and completely without changing what is said or adding information (transmission model) (Dysart-Gale 2007), and this role is being debated as too limiting for needs of clarification, patient advocacy, or the negotiation of cultural meanings or expectations in interpreted encounters (Brisset *et al.* 2013). Physician (Rosenberg *et al.* 2007) and interpreter (Rosenberg *et al.* 2008) perceptions of the process differ. A survey of 619 doctors and medical students (Hudelson *et al.* 2012) found that over half felt highly competent in working with interpreters, though some could not identify best practices in response to a vignette.

8.3 Method

Rationale for the sample

This qualitative study is intended to generate hypotheses for future testing, and uses a convenience sample. The site was chosen because a one-year chart review of pregnant women involved in routine prenatal care identified a disparity in a common marker of quality prenatal care, in that Hispanic women at the selected clinic were noted to have a higher incidence of urinary tract infections than Black or White women. Since urinary tract infections occur more frequently in pregnancy, particularly during the second and third trimester, physicians were expected to order a urinalysis test and inquire about reported symptoms or risks – a process that requires communication.

Women were approached in the prenatal clinic of the tertiary care hospital and invited to participate in a study comparing communication, decision making, and quality of care between Spanish-speaking Hispanics and English speakers (Table 8.1). A series of 16 prenatal encounters between physicians, medical interpreters, and patients were recorded during 2006 and 2007, to generate potential patterns for study. The original

Table 8.1 Preliminary descriptive comparison of visits.

Patient	**Number of words**			**Minutes**
	Total	**Physician**	**Patient**	
English-speaker	707	509 (72%)	198 (28%)	10:00
Spanish-speaker with interpreter	710	523 (74%)	187 (26%)	12:07

recordings varied in quality and some were eliminated when word units could not be counted or understood. All women in the study were seen during routine prenatal visits in the second and third trimester and had been seen previously by the same physicians. All the Spanish speakers were from Mexico, and they used a qualified hospital interpreter to speak with their physician. The same physician was then recorded discussing a similar prenatal agenda with a patient who spoke English as her primary (L1) language (four Black women and four White women). All interpreters in the study followed the transmission model of interpretation (Dysart-Gale 2007), which was part of the hospital requirement. The six physicians were second- and third-year residents in obstetrics/gynecology (four men and two women), all of whom were L1 English speakers. The study was approved by the Institutional Review Board (IRB) of the affiliated university, with informed consent in English and Spanish.

All recordings were transcribed word for word, with the translations from Spanish to English in-text. In review of transcriptions for variations in length and word count, the interpreter sequences were eliminated to compare physician–patient ratios of talk. Whether L1 English speakers or Spanish speakers with LEP, the patients received roughly the same amount of words in discussions with physicians and participated for only a quarter of the time. This particular equity in service reflects a physician's dominant control of communication in traditional obstetrics, which is also well documented in other specialties (Cordella 2004; Peck and Denney 2012). Interpreted encounters averaged about two minutes more, but the presence of the interpreter did not permit more patient participation or additional information exchange with the physician. Though this small sample does not permit inferences, the pattern merits further study and a larger sample size.

Comparison of discursive practices and shared decision making

Transcriptions were reviewed in two ways. First, each transcription was examined using discourse analysis (Jones 2018), with a focus on what Johnstone (2018) describes as discourse structure, i.e. the parts and sequences that make up the patterns in a co-constructed dialogue and the speech acts that signal intentions and ways of making meaning. Using this approach, the focus is on the highly ritualized prenatal visit as a genre, the framing of the encounter at the beginning, the types of questions asked, and how stories are generated. A matrix was established for each of these discourse practices and the transcriptions categorized for English and LEP speakers. For example, questions were sorted into yes/no, direct/close-ended, and open-ended types, and interruptions were grouped, following Goldberg (1990) as rapport building, neutral, or power oriented and so on. Although previous analysis of bilingual visits in medical encounters found interpreters often did not relay patient questions as asked (Davidson 2001), the interpreters in this series echoed questions systematically.

Both monolingual and bilingual encounters were also rated using an established and reliable tool to identify potential variations in shared decision making linked to language: the OPTION shared decision making scale (Elwyn *et al.* 2005; Melbourne *et al.* 2010).The OPTION scale includes 12 items, rated in terms of magnitude from 0 (none) to 4 (highest), for clinician behaviors. The following data analysis suggests that five discursive practices (question patterns, context cues from the lifeworld, any stories generated, humor, and attention to emotion cues) and the magnitude of shared decision-making scores may differ in interpreted encounters.

8.4 Data analysis

Discourse analysis approach to categorizing practices

The 16 transcriptions were coded systematically, but could not be stripped of investigator knowledge of L1 or LEP status: even with the interpreter text removed, particular phrases of both physician and patient could identify LEP encounters. For example, despite medical center staff and resident orientation by the Office of Interpreter Services that included instructions to use the first person and speak directly to the second language patient, there were instances when this practice did not occur, as seen in Excerpt 1.

Excerpt 1

Dr: Tell her we're getting very close. I actually saw them yesterday or 2 days ago?

In the above example, the physician directs the interpreter to provide a message to the patient using third person (line 1), yet uses the pronoun 'we', positioning the physician and patient together in awaiting the birth. A side conversation with the interpreter then takes place in which the use of 'them' positions the Hispanic family as separate from the two speakers, which is not interpreted.

Patterns of questions in medical discourse

Particular types of questions in institutional settings such as medical encounters position the primary speaker or physician as more powerful, provide for the distribution of turns in ways that set appropriate roles, and set up question-and-answer sequences that establish differing levels of participation and information exchange (Ehrlich and Freed 2010). To determine whether questions in this selected prenatal setting followed typical patterns documented in medical encounters (Heritage 2010), a matrix was constructed sorting questions into physician-initiated yes/no questions, close-ended direct questions, open-ended questions, and patient-initiated questions. Table 8.2 summarizes the pattern of questions during the prenatal visits with both LEP and L1 English-speaking pregnant women and their physicians. Though many of the questions for both groups were brief and predominantly solicited agreement, a pattern emerges of more open-ended questions and patient-initiated questions with L1 speakers.

In all the visits with Spanish-speaking patients and their interpreters, the physician uses the question design to set a medical agenda of problem definition and pregnancy surveillance that is highly structured. By contrast, in interactions with the English-speaking patients, the increase in open-ended questions provides more opportunity for patients to initiate an agenda item, request more clarification, and participate a bit more, and for the physicians to provide more details. In Excerpts 2 and 3, the construction of questions involves patients with gestational diabetes differently in discussing their diets.

Table 8.2 Comparison of questions.

Patient	Questions			
	Yes/no	Direct	Open-ended	Patient-Initiated
LEP 1	8	1	1	1
LEP 2	10	1	1	1
LEP 3	16	1	1	1
LEP 4	22	1	1	2
LEP 5	9	2	2	1
LEP 6	13	1	1	0
LEP 7	9	1	0	4
LEP 8	3	0	0	2
Average	11.3	1	1	1.5
L1 English 1	14	2	2	4
L1 English 2	11	2	2	3
L1 English 3	13	1	2	2
L1 English 4	33	10	4	2
L1 English 5	7	5	4	1
L1 English 6	19	1	3	6
L1 English 7	9	0	1	4
L1 English 8	9	1	2	10
Average	14.4	2.8	2.5	4

Excerpt 2: (from LEP #4)

Dr: OK? The other reason is that you have diabetes of
pregnancy, gestational diabetes.
Int.: La otra razón es porque tiene diabetes del
embarazo.
Pt: Mmm-hmm.
Dr: How are you doing with that?
Int.: ¿Qué tal lo lleva?
Pt: Mmmmm.....estoy teniendo una dieta y
pinchadome de estas para estar comiendo
verduras, frutas.
Int.: I have a diet that I've been on, and I've been the
finger sticks, and eating vegetables and fruits.
Dr: Good. Now, ummm, did you bring your finger
stick blood sugar log? There it is....
Pt: Sí.

In Excerpt 2, the physician asks an open-ended question in line 6 that allows the Hispanic patient to respond with positive agency for one sentence about a diet she has been maintaining to manage her diabetes and monitor her sugar. Instead of pursuing this cue embedded in the patient's lifeworld, in line 14 the physician responds with an evaluation and a change of subject that ends any discussion of what type of diet the patient is following. The practice described in education research by Mehan (1979) as initiation-response-evaluation (IRE) occurs: the physician expert poses a question, awaits the correct response, and then provides a positive reward that the patient has responded as expected, and moves on. This type of interaction question design involves little opportunity for participation or the exploration or exchange of information.

In Table 8.2, the Hispanic woman whose encounter has the most patient-initiated questions (LEP 7, with four) is accompanied by her mother and they apologize for asking so many questions. In an exit interview, they explain that this interpreter, who is an Anglo second-language Spanish speaker, is kind to them, whereas the usual interpreter assigned to the clinic and that they have had previously is an L1 Spanish speaker from another country who does not like Mexicans and discourages extra time or questions.

By contrast, in Excerpt 3 the patient responds to an unclear opening query about a glucose value and diet in an exchange that demonstrates more mutual participation.

Excerpt 3: (from L1 #3)

Pt: ...Rice Krispies and Honey Combs is like 1 ½ cup.
Dr: Yeah, that's a lot of carbs though, so that might be, that might be it. Yeah
Pt: Yeah, I'm gonna try – do something not as high in carbs.
Dr: Eggs – low carbs and good protein
Pt: Cereals are so much quicker.
Dr: I know it is.
Pt: ... Get out the front door, here bus comes at like 6:40.
Dr: Yeah.
Pt: I mean I can cut back to maybe 1 cup and try that?
Dr: It's still gonna be a lot of carbs.
Pt: Oh, OK.
Dr: OK its carbs, so you're gonna be really high there,

17 so anything you could do to cut that back would
18 probably be good. Try and do something else for
19 breakfast. You can always do hard-boiled eggs
20 the night before. Save a lot of time so you have a
21 couple of mornings worth of breakfast waiting for
22 you. And you know, do a banana and some sort of
23 fruit with that and you get a little carbs but not a
24 whole lot.
25 Pt: Right.
26 Dr: And certainly a lot less than – a serving of like
27 Honey Combs.
28 Pt: OK.

In this interaction, the patient describes the cereal she eats in line 1. The physician's correction begins with a 'Yeah' affirmation rather than a negative, which the patient echoes in line 4, signaling a joint problem-solving, shared decision-making sequence where suggestions, patient preferences, and alternatives are offered, weighed, and accepted in lines 19 and 21. When the patient suggests a compromise in lines 12 and 13, the physician provides a reminder rather than a rejection, and then an echo sequence follows of 'OK' in lines 15 and 16 that allow the negotiation of agreement. The interaction also shows a shared indexicality that rarely appears in the LEP interactions, reflecting L1 speech partners who are familiar with the same cereal and acknowledge that buses come early, and the physician positions suggestions in the patient's home and lifeworld through lines 16–24.

Involvement of the lifeworld

In considering how medical discourse may construct either humane care or narrow biomedical agendas, Mishler (1984) refers to the tendency of physicians to frame their questions and instructions within a technical agenda and neglect the patients' concerns and references to their condition within their daily lives, which he referred to as their lifeworld. Another difference between the English L1 interviews and the LEP interviews were that the latter had few preliminaries, few references to the patient's lifeworld, and not much rapport-building or joking sequences. In the interactions with English speakers, most interactions begin with a segment not predominantly biomedical, as shown in Excerpt 4

Excerpt 4: (from L1 #5)

Dr: You work at Burger King? Which one?
Pt: On Aviation. You been to that one?
Dr: Yeah, I've been to that one a lot, down the street from the Popeye's.
Pt: I work the drive-thru.
Dr: Oh, you do?
Pt: And then, I'm trying to work.... *(interruption)*
Nurse: We've been working to get her to be able to sit down because her legs hurt her after a full long day shift.
Dr: That sounds fair.
Pt: Yeah, I goes to work from 5 o'clock and gets off like 2 o'clock.
Dr: Yeah

In this L1 interaction, the obstetric visit begins with a connection with the patient's lifeworld and rapport building. The common indexicality in line 2, the patient's reference to a shared recognition of the same fast food restaurant in 'that one', and the physician's acknowledgment of 'that one' in line 3, create a shared experience and indexical ground outside biomedicine. In this segment, the patient has an opportunity to set the topic of work which the physician shifts in four subsequent turns to managing her blood sugar. Later in the same visit, the physician and the nurse negotiate an appointment, bringing in the lifeworld of the university medical center and a planned graduation that will disrupt traffic that they are trying to help the patient avoid.

By contrast, the LEP interviews in this sample start with a medical question about past pregnancy loss, fetal kick counts, or blood sugar checks. Pregnant Hispanic women who are LEP and new to the area in which the medical center is located are twice as likely as Whites to live below the poverty line (South Carolina Office of Rural Health 2006; US Census Bureau 2017), are more likely to live in sub-standard housing and lack health insurance, to have problems with public safety as a vulnerable population with language barriers in the community, and to lack access to public or private transportation (Young 2005; Cooper-Lewter 2013) – a situation that has changed little over the last decade. Despite these disparities, though physicians asked the global '*Any problems?*' question to LEP women with interpreters, none in the transcribed encounters were asked about living or working conditions, family or house members, access to transportation, food availability, or dimensions of their social lives and lifeworld, nor did the women respond with other than prompted biomedical issues.

Humor as a discursive practice

The use of humor in patient–physician interactions has been associated with better patient outcomes (Beck *et al.* 2002) and decreased malpractice claims (Levinson *et al.* 1997). Though humor may have a positive effect on such interactions, recent evidence suggests that social status markers matter and physicians may use humor differently with those they perceive of lower socioeconomic status (Haskard Zolnierek *et al.* 2009; McCreaddie and Payne 2014). There are few instances of joking or humor in the eight prenatal visits with women who are characterized as LEP. In one of the three identifiable moments of physician or family-member laughter, the Hispanic woman and the interpreter are not heard to respond. In Excerpt 5, the physician has been following up the pregnant woman's history of three previous miscarriages with a rhetoric of normalization of losing pregnancies.

Excerpt 5: (from LEP #5)

Dr: And I know that miscarriages are really hard.
Int.: Y sabemos que un malparto siempre es muy difícil.
Dr: But right now you have a very healthy active baby inside of you.
Int.: Pero ahora mismo usted tiene un bebé muy saludable y activo dentro.
Dr: I measured his size and he's growing perfectly.
Int.: Y le hemos medido el tamaño y está creciendo normalmente.
Dr: So I very much hope and think that this is going to turn into a baby that you get to take home.
Int.: Entonces yo pienso que esto se va a convertir en un bebé que usted puede llevar a casa.
Dr: OK? *(laughs)*
(silence)
Dr: Umm, today we're going to have to get some bloodwork from you.
Int.: Que hoy le vamos a sacar una muestras de sangre.

Whether the source of the humor that prompts the physician's laughter in line 15 is emotional discomfort, a facial expression, or some cognitive imagery regarding turning a belly (referred to as 'this') into a baby cannot be determined by the text – there were no exit interviews conducted with physicians. The sequence has the earlier, first topic of three pregnancy losses re-introduced with line 1's link to claim the conversational floor, 'And', accompanied by reassurance that allows the patient no opportunity to express emotion or join the conversation as the interpreter provides interpretation. The physician asserts agency for the pregnancy in lines 4–5 and 8, for work in monitoring the baby and for turning it back to the patient's charge after his work is done. The physician's laughter prompts no patient response and a silence follows. The clinician then repairs with a commissive that positions the physician and institution as 'we' and the patient again as 'you', a plan not offered for discussion or shared decision making.

The second instance of humor is shown in Excerpt 6, which takes place midway through a different LEP encounter.

Excerpt 6: (from LEP #2)

1 Int.: You're not taking any medicines for your diabetes,
2 right?
3 Pt. no
4 Dr: no, great *(in English)*
5 Int.: *(in English)* It's cold in this room
6 Dr: *(laughs)* I know
7 Dr: Overall these look very good
8 Int.: Overall these look very good
9 Pt: Mm-hm

The interpreter initiates a joke sequence with the physician, but does not interpret it with the patient, a move that leaves the patient without understanding for the humor sequence unless the non-verbals acted as cues. No laughter is heard from the patient. Several speaking turns later during the physical exam, the joke continues, without patient participation, as shown in Excerpt 7.

Excerpt 7: (from LEP #2)

1 Loud noise stops, rustling of paper
2 Dr: I am freezing
3 Int.: and with your belly out *(in English)*

Dr: *(laughing)* I'm just going to measure you real fast
Int.: Going to measure you rapidly
(interprets line 5)

The final laugh sequence in the total LEP sample happens Excerpt 8, when the husband (Part.), who speaks some English), conducts a side conversation with the physician not interpreted for the patient.

Excerpt 8: (from LEP #7)

Dr: Good, she's doing really well. The big thing
right now is if you have a big gush of clear fluid
like water, or if you have vaginal bleeding or if you
have contractions 5 minutes apart, you need to
come in. Also if she's not feeling the baby move.
Part.: So just a few days then – couple of weeks?
(laughter)
Dr: I can't predict that.
Part.: She doesn't want to go to the store, she says what
happens if I have the baby in the store?
Dr: *(unclear)* her first baby she'll probably be in early
labor for 24–48 hours. So you can go to the store.
Part.: What happens if her water breaks in the store?
Dr: Even if her water breaks she'll have plenty of time
to get to the hospital.
Part.: She'll have to pick him up off the floor and wipe
him off *(laughs)*.

The physician's use of pronoun positions the patient as an excluded third person, yet in lines 2–4 there is a shift to the second person 'you' to refer to bleeding and contractions that the patient may experience, not the husband. The husband introduces the uncertainty of waiting as a barrier to his wife's desire to go to the store in lines 9–10, culminating in the joke not shared in lines 16–17.

By contrast, all but one of the L1 transcriptions contain a humor element shared between the patient and physician, without the filter of an interpreter or a non-interpreting family member. Excerpt 9 is an example of this.

Excerpt 9: (from L1 #1)

Dr: Yeah, um you need um, you need alternatives for
birth control after you *[= (interruption)*
Pt: I'm not taking birth control. I'm getting my tubes

4 tied.
5 Dr: Have you signed papers or anything like that?
6 Pt: Yeah.
7 Dr: Great.
8 Pt: I'm getting my tubes tied *(unclear, exaggerated tone)*
9 Dr: Alright, no more!
10 Pt: I don't need no more babies! *(laughs)*
11 Dr: No more!
12 Pt: I'm getting too old for that.
13 Nurse: *(laughs)* All right!

The L1 patient initiates an interruption of the physician in line 3, a discursive practice not seen in the LEP encounters, where the Hispanic women did not claim the conversational floor so assertively. The repetition in lines 3–4 and 8, with exaggeration, echoes Tannen's (2007) observations that such practices provide the basis for connection during interaction as the speech partners take up the repeated cue. The laughter and exaggeration allow the physician and nurse to ratify their participation and listening, with two word echoes in lines 11 and 13 and an affirmation in line 13. The recognition of the shared language phrase 'no more' would have been less possible with an interpreter, nor did the shared indexical ground of such joking occur in LEP encounters.

In Excerpt 10, a pre-closing sequence has the physician changing his mind and deciding to check the patient's cervix for signs of imminent labor.

Excerpt 10: (from L1 #2)

1 Dr: Um, we're going to check your cervix.
2 Pt: OK!
3 Dr: Alright you look like you're ready, you're
4 prepared.
5 *(laughter)*
6 OK, let me grab one of the nurses and we will do
7 that. I'm gonna leave you an extra sheet there.
8 Pt: OK.
9 *(shared laughter)*

The physician's introduced topic in line 1 is welcomed by the patient, who is tired of being pregnant (an earlier theme), and she gladly agrees in line 2. The physician accepts her enthusiastic response as potential labor readiness in lines 3–4. The informal rhetoric of 'grab one of the nurses' and 'I'm gonna leave you' establishes a basis for connection and a foundation for the shared humor.

Though there are other examples of humor in the other L1 interactions, two others reveal the social play that these L1 joking sequences share, often based on exaggeration or poking gentle fun at particular elements of the pregnancy-based medical encounter. In the L1 interactions, the pregnant woman helps to generate or maintain the connection using language to moderate stress or build intimacy, unlike in the LEP encounters.

In Excerpt 11, as the encounter ends with a physician's pre-closing sequence, a non-response in line 2 triggers a humor sequence.

Excerpt 11: (from L1 #4)

Dr: Ah, do you have any questions or concerns today?
Pt: Um, no.
Dr: Anything you wanna talk about? Weather,
politics, sports?
Pt: *(laughs)*
Dr: Barry Bonds, President Bush spying on you
making phone calls?
Pt: No.
Dr: No one wants to talk about any of that today. I
don't really know anything about it anyway, I was
just checking.
Pt: *(laughs)*
Dr: All right, well we'll see ya, ok, um, lets do 2
weeks, okay? You have any problems you let us
know alright?
Pt: I certainly will.
Dr: All right __*(unclear)* let her get her shoes now.
Pt: *(laughs)*

The topics that the physician introduces as utterances in lines 3–4 are playful, since the frames they represent fall far outside the expected frame of the medical encounter. When the physician returns to the topic of continuing medical surveillance in lines 13–14, the patient responds positively 'I certainly will' as the laughter has re-energized her participation. The last joke in line 17 implies she has been held hostage, with resulting laughter at the absurdity.

Shared decision making with the OPTION Scale

Each of the medical encounters was coded using the OPTION Scale. Though the 12-question scale is rated with up to four points per response, little shared decision making took place according to the established criteria. The highly ritualized prenatal visit, in which most diagnostic surveillance and testing procedures are ordered rather than discussed or explained, resulted in relatively low scores overall for both groups, but they were lower for the Hispanic patients who had limited English proficiency and used interpreters (Table 8.3).

Table 8.3 Comparison of shared decision making: low for both groups, but lower for Hispanics.

	Mean
L1 English	10.5
Hispanics	4.4

Irrespective of primary language, there were few instances of the dimensions of shared decision making documented in the literature, such as soliciting the patient's agenda (Marvel *et al.* 1999) or building a history with the patient rather than taking it with a series of close-ended questions (Haidet and Paterniti 2003). Despite the relatively low scores, the level of shared decision making, while disappointing, does not differ too widely from that of other physicians faced with diagnoses considered confined by practice settings and involving visits shorter in duration, as seen in an example of depression visits in primary care (Young *et al.* 2008; Brenner *et al.* 2018).

8.5 Conclusion and implications

The patterns of questions suggest that physicians who use the predominantly yes/no question series narrowed the conversational floor and offered little opportunity for LEP patients to raise topics or initiate questions from their lifeworld. In exit interviews, patients acculturated to not interrupt or question the physician contributed to less participation, as did the intermediary role of the interpreter that offered less opportunity for connection. The unexpected finding of ethnic bias in one of the medical encounters between a family that perceived a barrier with an interpreter from another country suggests that social biases may be worth investigating in interpreter services. Finally, narrowed conversational floors, positioning that often excludes the LEP woman from full participation, and a prenatal ritual of sequential yes/no and close-ended questions based on surveillance and prescribed obstetric testing offered with few choices, all contribute to low levels of shared decision making in prenatal care overall, but especially for LEP women.

Since low levels of shared decision making are associated with poorer patient-reported health outcomes, higher healthcare use, and worse quality indicators (Hughes *et al.* 2018), recommendations to increase physician education regarding shared decision making should benefit prenatal care as well as other specialties, with a special focus on interpreted visits. Findings provide potential hypotheses for testing and descriptive evidence to support patient, provider, and interpreter training to enhance shared decision making in monolingual and bilingual encounters. In hopes of continuing improvement in care to persons with LEP, the US Department of Health and Human Services (DHHS) Office of Civil Rights issues a *Language Access Annual Progress Report* detailing active efforts to improve language assistance services, promote nondiscrimination in care to this population, and track efforts for change.1

Note

1 For the 2023 report see https://www.hhs.gov/sites/default/files/language-access-report-2023.pdf.

References

Aranguri, Cesar, Brad Davidson and Robert Ramirez (2006) Patterns of communication through interpreters: A detailed sociolinguistic analysis. *Journal of General Internal Medicine* 21 (6): 623–629. https://doi.org/10.1111/j.1525-1497.2006.00451.x

Balakrishnan, Vamsi, Jamie Roper, Kori Cossey, Crystal Roman and Rebecca Jeanmonod (2016) Misidentification of English language proficiency in triage: Impact on satisfaction and door-to-room time. *Journal of Immigrant & Minority Health* 18 (2): 369–373. https://doi.org/10.1007/s10903-015-0174-4

Beach, Mary C., Somnath Saha, P. Todd Korthuis, Victoria Sharp, Jonathon Cohn, Ira Wilson, Susan Eggly *et al.* (2010) Differences in patient–provider communication for Hispanic vs. non-Hispanic white patients in HIV care. *Journal of General Internal Medicine* 25 (7): 682–687. https://doi.org/10.1007/s11606-010-1310-4

Beach, Mary C., Jeremy Sugarman, Rachel L. Johnson, Jose J. Arbelaez, Patrick S. Duggan and Lisa A. Cooper (2005) Do patients treated with dignity report higher satisfaction, adherence, and receipt of preventive care? *Annals of Family Medicine* 3 (4): 3331–3338. https://doi.org/10.1370/afm.328

Beck, Rainer S., Rebecca Daughtridge and Philip D. Sloane (2002) Physician-patient communication in the primary care office: A systematic review. *Journal of the American Board of Family Medicine* 15 (1): 25–38.

Blay, Nicole, Sharelle Ioannou, Marika Seremetkoska, Jenny Morris, Gael Holters, Verily Thomas and Everett Bronwyn (2018) Healthcare interpreter utilisation: Analysis of health administrative data. *BMC Health Service Research* 18 (1): 348–354. https://doi.org/10.1186/s12913-018-3135-5

Brenner, Alison T., Teri L. Malo, Marjorie Margolis, Jennifer Elston Lafata, Shynah James, Maihan B. Vu and Daniel S. Reuland (2018) Evaluating shared decision making for lung cancer screening. *JAMA Internal Medicine* 178 (10): 1311–1316. https://doi.org/10.1001/jamainternmed.2018.3054

Brisset, Camille, Yvan Leanza and Karine Laforest (2013) Working with interpreters in health care: A systematic review and meta-ethnography of qualitative studies. *Patient Education & Counseling* 91 (2): 131–140. https://doi.org/10.1016/j.pec.2012.11.008

Brooks, Katherine, Bianca Stifani, Haiyan Ramírez Batlle, Maria Aguilera Nunez, Matthew Erlich and Joseph Diaz (2016) Patient perspectives on the need for and barriers to professional medical interpretation. *Rhode Island Medicine* 99 (1): 30–33.

Butow, Phyllis, Melanie Bell, David Goldstein, Ming Sze, Lynley Aldridge, Sarah Abdo, Michelle Mikhail *et al.* (2011) Grappling with cultural differences: Communication between oncologists and immigrant cancer patients with and without interpreters. *Patient Education & Counseling* 84 (3): 398–405. https://doi.org/10.1016/j.pec.2011.01.035

Carter-Pokras, Olivia, Marla J. F. O'Neill, Vasana Cheanvechai, Mikhail Menis, Tao Fan and Angelo Solera (2004). Providing linguistically appropriate services to persons with limited English proficiency: A needs and resources investigation. *American Journal of Managed Care* 10: SP29–SP36.

Chen, Alice Hm, Mara K. Youdelman and Jamie Brooks (2007) The legal framework for language access in healthcare settings: Title VI and beyond.

Journal of General Internal Medicine 22 (Suppl. 2): 362–367.

Cooper-Lewter, Stephanie K. (2013) *Research Brief: Latino Immigrant Families in South Carolina*. Columbia: Sisters of Charity Foundation of South Carolina. Available online: https://sistersofcharitysc.com/wp-content/uploads/2014/04/Research-Brief-March-2013.pdf

Cordella, Marisa (2004) *The Dynamic Consultation: A Discourse Analytical Study of Doctor–Patient Communication*. Amsterdam: John Benjamins. https://doi.org/10.1075/pbns.128

Davidson, Brad (2001) Questions in cross-linguistic medical encounters: The role of the hospital interpreter. *Anthropological Quarterly* 74 (4): 170–178. https://doi.org/10.1353/anq.2001.0035

Docherty, Angie, Carol Bugge and Andrew Watterson (2012) Engagement: An indicator of difference in the perceptions of antenatal care for pregnant women from diverse socioeconomic backgrounds. *Health Expectations* 15 (2): 126–138. https://doi.org/10.1111/j.1369-7625.2011.00684.x

Dysart-Gale, Deborah (2007) Clinicians and medical interpreters: Negotiating culturally appropriate care for patients with limited English ability. *Family and Community Health* 30 (3): 237–246. https://doi.org/10.1097/01.FCH.0000277766.62408.96

Elwyn, Glyn, Adrian Edwards and Rachel Thompson (eds) (2016) *Shared Decision Making in Health Care: Achieving Evidence-Based Patient Choice* (3rd edition). Oxford: Oxford University Press. https://doi.org/10.1093/acprof:oso/9780198723448.001.0001

Elwyn, Glyn, Hayley Hutchings, Adrian Edwards, Frances Rapport, Michel Wensing, Wai-Yee Cheung and Richard Grol (2005) The OPTION scale: Measuring the extent that clinicians involve patients in decision-making tasks. *Health Expectations* 8 (1): 34–42. https://doi.org/10.1111/j.1369-7625.2004.00311.x

Ehrlich, Susan and Alice Freed (2010) The function of questions in institutional discourse. In Alice Freed and Susan Ehrlich (eds) *'Why Do You Ask?' The Function of Questions in Institutional Discourse*, 3–19. New York: Oxford University Press. https://doi.org/10.1093/acprof:oso/9780195306897.003.0001

Fiscella, Kevin, Peter Franks, Mark P. Doescher and Barry Saver (2002) Disparities in health care by race, ethnicity, and language among the insured: Findings from a national sample. *Medical Care* 40 (1): 52–59. https://doi.org/10.1097/00005650-200201000-00007

Flynn, Sarah J., Lisa A. Cooper and Tiffany L. Gary-Webb (2014) The role of culture in promoting effective clinical communication, behavior change, and treatment adherence. In Leslie R. Martin and Robin DiMatteo (eds) *Communication, Behavior Change, and Treatment Adherence*,

167–185. Oxford: Oxford University Press. https://doi.org/10.1093/oxfordhb/9780199795833.013.020

Franks, Peter, Kevin Fiscella, Cleveland G. Shields, Sean C. Meldrum, Paul Duberstein, Anthony F. Jerant, Daniel J. Tancredi and Ronald M. Epstein (2005) Are patients' ratings of their physicians related to health outcomes? *Annals of Family Medicine* 3 (3): 229–234. https://doi.org/10.1370/afm.267

Goldberg, Julia A. (1990) Interrupting the discourse on interruptions: An analysis in terms of relationally neutral, power- and rapport-oriented acts. *Journal of Pragmatics* 14 (6): 883–903. https://doi.org/10.1016/0378-2166(90)90045-F

Haidet, Paul and Debora A. Paterniti (2003) 'Building' a history rather than 'taking' one: A perspective on information sharing during the medical interview. *Archives of Internal Medicine* 163 (10): 1134–1140. https://doi.org/10.1001/rchinte.163.10.1134

Haskard Zolnierek, Kelly B., M. Robin Dimatteo, Melissa M. Mondala, Zhou Zhang, Leslie R. Martin and Andrew H. Messiha (2009) Development and validation of the physician–patient humor rating scale. *Journal of Health Psychology* 14 (8): 1163–1173. https://doi.org/10.1177/1359105309342288

Haviland, Amelia M., Marc N. Elliott, Robert Weech-Maldonado, Katrin Hambarsoomian, Nate Orr and Ron D. Hays (2012) Racial/ethnic disparities in Medicare Part D experiences. *Medical Care* 50 (Suppl.): S40–S47. https://doi.org/10.1097/MLR.0b013e3182610aa5

Heritage, John (2010) Questioning in medicine. In Alice F. Freed and Susan Ehrlich (eds) *'Why Do You Ask?' The Function of Questions in Institutional Discourse*, 42–68. New York: Oxford University Press.

Hsieh, Elaine (2006) Understanding medical interpreters: Reconceptualizing bilingual communication. *Health Communication* 20 (2): 177–186. https://doi.org/10.1207/s15327027hc2002_9

Hudelson, Patricia, Thomas Perneger, Véronique Kolly and Noëlle J. Perron (2012) Self-assessed competency at working with a medical interpreter is not associated with knowledge of good practice. *PLoS One* 7 (6): e38973. https://doi.org/10.1371/journal.pone.0038973

Hughes, Tasha M., Katiuscha Merath, Qinyu Chen, Steven Sun, Elizabeth Palmer, Jay J. Idrees, Victor Okunrintemi *et al.* (2018) Association of shared decision-making on patient-reported health outcomes and healthcare utilization. *American Journal of Surgery* 216 (1): 7–12. https://doi.org/10.1016/j.amjsurg.2018.01.011

Jiang, Lihua, Chong Han, Jinlin Jiang and Yue Feng (2014) The sociological turn in the interpreter's role: Discourse interpreting filters. *Translation and Interpreting Studies* 9 (2): 274–298. https://doi.org/10.1075/tis.9.2.07jia

Johnstone, Barbara (2018) *Discourse Analysis* (3rd edition). Hoboken, NJ: John Wiley.

Jones, Rodney H. (2018). Discourse and health communication. In Deborah Tannen, Heidi E. Hamilton and Deborah Schiffrin (eds) *The Handbook of Discourse Analysis* (2nd edition), 841–856. Oxford: John Wiley / Blackwell. https://doi.org/10.1002/9781118584194.ch39

Kamara, Daniella, Jon Weil, Janey Youngblom, Claudia Guerra and Galen Joseph (2018) Cancer counseling of low-income limited English proficient Latina women using medical interpreters: Implications for shared decision-making. *Journal of Genetic Counseling* 27 (1): 155–168. https://doi.org/10.1007/s10897-017-0132-5

Karliner, Leah S., Elizabeth A. Jacobs, Alice Hm Chen and Sunita Mutha (2007) Do professional interpreters improve clinical care for patients with limited English proficiency? A systematic review of the literature. *Health Service Research* 42 (2): 727–754. https://doi.org/10.1111/j.1475-6773.2006.00629.x

Kirkham, Colleen, Susan Harris and Stefan Grzybowski (2005) Evidence-based prenatal care: Part I. General prenatal care and counseling issues. *American Family Physician* 71 (7): 1264–1266.

Kuntz, Jennifer L., Monika M. Safford, Jasvinder A.Singh, Shobha Phansalkar, Sarah P. Slight, Qoua Liang Her, Nancy Allen Lapointe *et al.* (2014) Patient-centered interventions to improve medication management and adherence: A qualitative review of research findings. *Patient Education & Counseling* 97 (3): 310–326. https://doi.org/10.1016/j.pec.2014.08.021

Leanza, Yvan, Isabelle Boivin and Ellen Rosenberg (2010) Interruptions and resistance: A comparison of medical consultations with family and trained interpreters. *Social Science & Medicine* 70 (12): 1888–1895. https://doi.org/10.1016/j.socscimed.2010.02.036

Levinson, Wendy, Debra L. Roter, John P. Mullooly, Valerie T. Dull and Richard M. Frankel (1997) Physician-patient communication: The relationship with malpractice claims among primary care physicians and surgeons. *Journal of the American Medical Association* 277 (7): 553–559. https://doi.org/10.1001/jama.1997.03540310051034

Lindholm, Mary, J. Lee Hargraves, Warren J. Ferguson and George Reed (2012) Professional language interpretation and inpatient length of stay and readmission rates. *Journal of General Internal Medicine* 27 (10): 1294–1299. https://doi.org/10.1007/s11606-012-2041-5

Little, Paul, Hazel Everitt, Ian Williamson, Greg Warner, Michael Moore, Clare Gould, Kate Ferrier and Sheila Payne (2001) Observational study of patient-centeredness and positive approach on outcomes of general practice consultations. *British Medical Journal* 323 (7318): 908–911. https://doi.org/10.1136/bmj.323.7318.908

Marvel, M. Kim, Ronald M. Epstein, Kristine Flowers and Howard B. Beckman (1999) Soliciting the patient's agenda: Have we improved? *Journal of the American Medical Association* 281 (3): 283–287. https://doi.org/10.1001/jama.281.3.283

McCreaddie, May and Sheila Payne (2014) Humour in health-care interactions: A risk worth taking. *Health Expectations* 17 (3): 332–344. https://doi.org/10.1111/j.1369-7625.2011.00758.x

Mehan, Hugh (1979) *Learning Lessons: Social Organization in the Classroom.* Cambridge, MA: Harvard University Press. https://doi.org/10.4159/harvard.9780674420106

Melbourne, Emma, Kate Sinclair, Marie-Anne Durand, France Légaré and Glyn Elwyn (2010) Developing a dyadic OPTION scale to measure perceptions of shared decision making. *Patient Education & Counseling* 78 (2): 177–183. https://doi.org/10.1016/j.pec.2009.07.009

Menendez, Mariano E., Markus Loeffler and David Ring (2015) Patient satisfaction in an outpatient hand surgery office: A comparison of English- and Spanish-speaking patients. *Quality Management in Health Care* 24 (4): 183–189. https://doi.org/10.1097/QMH.0000000000000074

Mishler, Elliot (1984) *The Discourse of Medicine: Dialectics of Medical Interviews.* Norwood, NJ: Ablex Publishing.

Morales, Leo S., Steve P. Reise and Ron D. Hays (2000) Evaluating the equivalence of care ratings by Whites and Hispanics. *Medical Care* 38 (5): 517–527. https://doi.org/10.1097/00005650-200005000-00008

National Board of Certification for Medical Interpreters (2016a) *Certified Medical Interpreter Candidate Handbook.* Available online: https://nbcmi.memberclicks.net/assets/docs/national-board-candidate-handbook.pdf

National Board of Certification for Medical Interpreters (2016b) *2016 Annual Report.* Available online: https://nbcmi.memberclicks.net/assets/docs/nbcmi%20annual%20report%202016%20final.pdf

Ngo-Metzger, Quyen, Dara H. Sorkin, Russell S. Phillips, Sheldon Greenfield, Michael P. Massagli, Brian Clarridge and Sherrie H. Kaplan (2007) Providing high-quality care for limited English proficient patients: The importance of language concordance and interpreter use. *Journal of General Internal Medicine* 22 (Suppl. 2): 324–330. https://doi.org/10.1007/s11606-007-0340-z

Nieuwenhuijze, Marianne, Irene Korstjens, Ank de Jonge, Raymond de Vries and Antoine Lagro-Janssen (2014) On speaking terms: A Delphi study on shared decision-making in maternity care. *BMC Pregnancy & Childbirth* 14: 223. https://doi.org/10.1186/1471-2393-14-223

Njeru, Jane W., Deborah H. Boehm, Debra J. Jacobson, Laura M. Guzman-Corrales, Chun Fan, Scott Shimotsu and Mark L. Wieland (2017) Diabetes outcome and process measures among patients who require language interpreter services in Minnesota primary care practices. *Journal of Community Health* 42 (4): 819–825. https://doi.org/10.1007/s10900-017-0323-x

October, Tessie W., Pamela Hinds, Jichuan Wang, Zoelle B. Dizon, Yao Cheng and Debra Roter (2016) Parent satisfaction with communication is associated with physician's patient-centered communication patterns during family conferences. *Pediatric Critical Care Medicine* 17 (6): 490–497. https://doi.org/10.1097/PCC.0000000000000719

Palmer, Nynikka R. A., Erin E. Kent, Laura P. Forsythe, Neeraj K. Arora, Julia H. Rowland, Noreen M. Aziz, Danielle Blanch-Hartigan *et al.* (2014) Racial and ethnic disparities in patient-provider communication, quality-of-care ratings, and patient activation among long-term cancer survivors. *Journal of Clinical Oncology* 32 (36): 4087–4094. https://doi.org/10.1200/JCO.2014.55.5060

Peck, B. Mitchell and Meredith Denney (2012) Disparities in the conduct of the medical encounter: The effects of physician and patient race and gender. *SAGE Open* 2 (3): 1–14. https://doi.org/10.1177/2158244012459193

Phillips, Christine B. and Joanne Travaglia (2011) Low levels of uptake of free interpreters by Australian doctors in private practice: Secondary analysis of national data. *Australian Health Review* 35 (4): 475–479. https://doi.org/10.1071/AH10900

Plewnia, Anne, Jürgen Bengel and Mirjam Körner (2016) Patient-centeredness and its impact on patient satisfaction and treatment outcomes in medical rehabilitation. *Patient Education & Counseling* 99 (12): 2063–2070. https://doi.org/10.1016/j.pec.2016.07.018

Rivadeneyra, Rocio, Virginia Elderkin-Thompson, Roxane Cohen Silver and Howard Waitzkin (2000) Patient-centeredness in medical encounters requiring an interpreter. *American Journal of Medicine* 108 (6): 470–474. https://doi.org/10.1016/S0002-9343(99)00445-3

Roberts, Celia, Becky Moss, Val Wass, Srikant Sarangi and Roger Jones (2005) Misunderstandings: A qualitative study of primary care consultations in multilingual settings, and educational implications. *Medical Education* 39 (5): 465–475. https://doi.org/10.1111/j.1365-2929.2005.02121.x

Rosenberg, Ellen, Yvan Leanza and Robbyn Seller (2007) Doctor–patient communication in primary care with an interpreter: Physician perceptions of professional and family interpreters. *Patient Education & Counseling* 67 (3): 286–292. https://doi.org/10.1016/j.pec.2007.03.011

Rosenberg, Ellen, Robbyn Seller and Yvan Leanza (2008) Through interpreters' eyes: Comparing roles of professional and family interpreters. *Patient Education Counseling* 70 (1): 87–93. https://doi.org/10.1016/j.pec.2007.09.015

Saville-Troike, Muriel (2003) *The Ethnography of Communication: An Introduction* (3rd edition). Malden, MA: Blackwell. https://doi.org/10.1002/9780470758373

Schegloff, Emanuel A. (2007) *Sequence Organization in Interaction: A Primer in Conversation Analysis, Volume 1.* Cambridge: Cambridge University Press. https://doi.org/10.1017/CBO9780511791208

Schouten, Barbara C. and Ludwien Meeuwesen (2006) Cultural differences in medical communication: A review of the literature. *Patient Education and Counseling* 64 (1–3): 21–34. https://doi.org/10.1016/j.pec.2005.11.014

Schwei, Rebecca J., Sam Del Pozo, Niels Agger-Gupta, Wilma Alvarado-Little, Ann Bagchi, Alice Hm Chen, Lisa Diamond *et al.* (2016) Changes in research on language barriers in health care since 2003: A cross-sectional review study. *International Journal of Nursing Studies* 54: 36–44. https://doi.org/10.1016/j.ijnurstu.2015.03.001

Seale, Clive, Carol Rivas and Moira Kelly (2013) The challenge of communication in interpreted consultations in diabetes care: A mixed methods study. *British Journal of General Practice* 63 (607): e125–e133. https://doi.org/10.3399/bjgp13X663082

Sentell, Tetine and Kathryn L. Braun (2012) Low health literacy, limited English proficiency, and health status in Asians, Latinos, and other racial/ethnic groups in California. *Journal of Health Communication* 17 (Suppl. 3): 82–99. https://doi.org/10.1080/10810730.2012.712621

Smith, Diane L. (2010) Health care disparities for persons with limited English proficiency: Relationships from the 2006 Medical Expenditure. Panel Survey (MEPS). *Journal of Health Disparities Research and Practice* 3 (Art. 4): 57–67. Available online: https://digitalscholarship.unlv.edu/jhdrp/vol3/iss3/4/

South Carolina Office of Rural Health (2006) *South Carolina Low Country Healthy Start Impact Report.* Available online: http://www.mchlibrary.info/mchbfinalreports/docs/h49mc00062.pdf

Suurmond, Jeanine and Conny Seeleman (2006) Shared decision-making in an intercultural context: Barriers in the interaction between physicians and immigrant patients. *Patient Education and Counseling* 60 (2): 253–259. https://doi.org/10.1016/j.pec.2005.01.012

Tandon, S. Darius, Kathleen M. Parillo and Maureen Keefer (2005) Hispanic women's perceptions of patient-centeredness during prenatal care: A mixed methods study. *Birth* 32 (4): 312–317. https://doi.org/10.1111/j.0730-7659.2005.00389.x

Tannen, Deborah (2007) *Talking Voices. Repetition, Dialogue, and Imagery in Conversational Discourse* (2nd edition). Cambridge: Cambridge University Press. https://doi.org/10.1017/CBO9780511618987

Tucker Edmonds, Brownsyne (2014) Shared decision-making and decision support: Their role in obstetrics and gynecology. *Current Opinions in Obstetrics & Gynecology* 26 (6): 523–530. https://doi.org/10.1097/GCO.0000000000000120

US Agency for Healthcare Research and Quality (2017) *2016 National Healthcare Quality and Disparities Report*. Rockville, MD: Agency for Healthcare Research and Quality. AHRQ Publication 17-0001. Available online: https://archive.ahrq.gov/research/findings/nhqrdr/2014chartbooks/index.html

US Census Bureau (2017) Selected characteristics of people at specified levels of poverty in the past 12 months. 2012-2016 American Community Survey 5-year estimates. *American FactFinder*. Available online: https://factfinder.census.gov/faces/tableservices/jsf/pages/productview.xhtml?src=CF

US Department of Health and Human Services (2003) Guidance to Federal financial assistance recipients regarding Title VI Prohibition against national origin discrimination affecting limited English proficiency persons. *Federal Register* 68 (153): 47311–47322. Available online: https://www.govinfo.gov/content/pkg/FR-2003-08-08/pdf/03-20179.pdf

US Department of Health and Human Services (2013) *Language Access Plan 2013*. Washington, DC: US Department of Health and Human Services / Office for Civil Rights. Available online: https://www.hhs.gov/sites/default/files/hhs-language-access-plan2013.pdf

US Department of Health and Human Services (2016) 45 CFR Part 92: Nondiscrimination in health programs and activities. *Federal Register* 81 (96): 31376–31473. Available online: https://www.govinfo.gov/content/pkg/FR-2016-05-18/pdf/2016-11458.pdf

Van Cleave, Alisa C., Megan U. Roosen-Runge, Alison B. Miller, Lauren C. Milner, Katrina A. Karkazis, Katrina A. and David C. Magnus (2014) Quality of communication in interpreted versus non-interpreted PICU family meetings. *Critical Care Medicine* 42 (6): 1507–1517. https://doi.org/10.1097/CCM.0000000000000177

Weech-Maldonado, Robert, Marie N. Fongwa, Peter Gutierrez and Ron D. Hays (2008) Language and regional differences in evaluations of Medicare managed care by Hispanics. *Health Services Research* 43 (2): 552–568. https://doi.org/10.1111/j.1475-6773.2007.00796.x

Wilson-Stronks, Amy, Karen K. Lee, Christina L. Cordero, April L. Kopp and Erica Galvez (2008) *One Size Does not Fit All: Meeting the Health Care Needs of Diverse Populations.* Oakbrook Terrace, IL: The Joint Commission. Available online: http://www.jointcommission.org/assets/1/6/HLCOneSizeFinal.pdf

Young, Henry N., Robert A. Bell, Ronald M. Epstein, Mitchell D. Feldman and Richard L. Kravitz (2008) Physicians' shared decision-making behaviors in depression care. *Archives of Internal Medicine* 168 (13): 1404–1408. https://doi.org/10.1001/archinte.168.13.1404

Young, Richard D. (2005) *The Growing Hispanic Population in South Carolina: Trends and Issues.* Working Paper of the Institute for Public Service and Policy Research, University of South Carolina. Available online: http://www.ipspr.sc.edu/publication/Population%20In%20SC.pdf

Charlene Pope received her PhD in education with a focus on sociolinguistics from the University of Rochester and did a post-doctoral fellowship in preventive cardiology at the University of Rochester. She is Chief Nurse for Research at the Ralph H. Johnson Veterans Affairs (VA) Medical Center, and Affiliate Associate Professor at the Medical University of South Carolina College of Medicine Department of Pediatrics. Her research interests include the role of communication in health service disparities, patient–provider communication, and communication practices of older people of diverse ethnicities with and without Alzheimer's disease. Address for correspondence: Ralph H. Johnson VA Medical Center, 109 Bee Street, Rm. B249-D, Charleston, SC 29458, USA. Email: popec@musc.edu

Jason Roberson holds an MA in Spanish Linguistics from Pennsylvania State University, an MA in Hispanic Culture and Language from New York University, and an MDiv. from Virginia Theological Seminary. He previously worked at the Medical University of South Carolina as Coordinator of Interpreter Services and for the MUSC College of Nursing as grant coordinator of the Hispanic Health Initiative, funded by the Duke Endowment. He is an Episcopal priest and currently serves as Assistant Rector at Holy Cross Faith Memorial Episcopal Church in Pawleys Island, SC. Address for correspondence: 675 Blue Stem Drive, #71A Pawleys Island, SC 29585, USA. Email: jroberson@holycrossfm.org

9 Triadic medical interaction with a bilingual doctor

Louisa Willoughby, Marisa Cordella, Simon Musgrave & Julie Bradshaw

9.1 Introduction

As migration and globalization lead to increasingly diverse societies, communication issues in medical contexts become more complex. On the one hand this 'superdiversity' (Vertovec 2007) means medical professionals can expect to treat patients from a wide variety of language backgrounds, with health beliefs and levels of health literacy very different from those common in the wider society, as well as with varied competence in the majority language of the society (Fernandez *et al.* 2004; Sudore *et al.* 2009; O'Brien and Shea 2011). On the other hand, the increasing reliance on overseas medical graduates in countries like Australia, the UK and the US – together with migrant-background professionals who were trained in those countries – means that the medical workforce itself is increasingly multilingual.[1]

Multilingual practitioners may choose to communicate directly with migrant-background patients in a language other than that of the majority. Research from California, however, shows that in that state at least, the practice is widespread. A survey of over 1300 doctors and specialist physicians practising there found that 26% of primary-care and 22% of specialist physicians consulted in Spanish when required (Yoon *et al.* 2004: 127) while surveys and samples of Low English Proficiency medical patients regularly find that around 60–70% have a physician who speaks their native language (Wilson *et al.* 2005: 801; Masland *et al.* 2011). In Australia, the BEACH survey of general practitioners found that between 2006 and 2012 approximately 25% of surveyed GPs at least occasionally consulted in languages other than English (Britt *et al.* 2016: 23). Moreover, the survey found that around 3% of GPs conducted the majority of their consultations in one or more languages other than English (Britt *et al.* 2016: 23).

While the practice of doctors consulting in minority languages seems relatively common in the US and Australia at least, there has been little qualitative research on how such consultations unfold. Thus questions such as what role (if any) is played by English, how medical concepts and terminology are conveyed and the cause and resolution of any misunderstandings – have received scant attention (but see Vickers *et al.* 2015). In this article we start to answer these questions through a close analysis of interaction in one consultation which took place in Italian at an outpatients' clinic at a Melbourne hospital. As the patient was accompanied by her bilingual daughter, we also consider the role of the family member in the consultation, and how this role might be different from that played by family members in interpreted consultations. We did not actually set out to record language-concordant consultations, so we do not have other recordings for comparison. But since there is such a scarcity of qualitative research exploring communication in language-concordant medical consultations in languages other than English we offer our observations as a starting point that can hopefully be expanded on by researchers in the future (see Sarangi, this volume, for suggestions of how this line of research might unfold).

In this paper we first survey the literature on bilingual doctors and triadic consultations before introducing our data and methodology. Results begin with the dominant language frame, before considering the family member's role and the role of English in the consultation. General findings and implications are presented in the discussion and conclusion.

9.2 Bilingual doctors in the literature

In recent years there has been increasing research interest in outcomes for migrant patients who see a doctor who speaks their primary language, known as language-concordant physicians. These studies have been predominantly US-based and generally compare outcomes for those who saw a language-concordant physician against those of migrant patients who saw a language-discordant physician (e.g. an English monolingual doctor), either with or without the use of an interpreter. They show a general pattern of improved communication and health outcomes for those who see language-concordant physicians. For example, these patients report higher overall satisfaction (Ngo-Metzger *et al.* 2007; Dunlap *et al.* 2015), and are more likely to disclose use of complementary therapies (Chao *et al.* 2015), ask questions (Green *et al.* 2005) and rate their examiner's interpersonal communication skills highly (Baker *et al.* 1998). They are also less likely to have problems understanding a medical situation or medication labels or to have an adverse reaction to medications (Wilson *et al.* 2005). However, some of the advantages of seeing a language-concordant physician may also be gained by using professional interpreters in language-discordant consultations. In particular it seems that clinical outcomes – such as use of tests or comprehension of a treatment plan – may be similar between the two groups (Hampers and McNulty 2002; Fernandez *et al.* 2004), although patients' reported level of overall satisfaction varies from study to study (Lee *et al.* 2002; Dunlap *et al.* 2015). Such findings invite us to look more closely at the practices within individual language-concordant consultations to better understand the processes that seem to be leading to improved patient rapport.

The consulting practices of bilingual doctors are also of interest because – unlike professional interpreters – they are not required to complete specialist training or certification before consulting in a minority language.[2] While many may have completed their medical training in the minority language before migrating to the country where they are now certified to practice, the literature makes clear that a number of Spanish-speaking language-concordant health professionals in the US at least are second-language speakers, and this may impact their ability to communicate effectively with patients (Fernandez *et al.* 2004; Yoon *et al.* 2004; Vickers *et al.* 2015). Doctors practising in a migrant language may also have to negotiate complex linguistic terrain, such as when a patient or family member uses some English in the consultation and the doctor must decide in which language to respond. While statistical studies suggest language-concordant medical professionals communicate well with their patients on average, we should expect varied competencies from professional to professional. This is partially borne out by the only study to date (that we are aware of) that conducts a discourse analysis of a language-concordant consultation: Vickers *et al.* (2015) looked at the code-switching behaviour of two nurses bilingual in English and Spanish at a low-income clinic in California in consultations involving a family member. They found that the family members frequently code-switched to English, causing problems for the nurses, who often responded in

English and thus excluded the patient from the discourse (a common issue in multiparty interpreted consultations that is also discussed by Sarangi and also by Roberts and Sarangi, this volume).

There are many complex factors influencing the efficacy of interpreted and language-concordant consultations, including the setting, reason for consultation, patient's health literacy and the linguistic skills and communication training of all parties involved. In this article, it is not our intention to assess language-concordant consultations in comparison with those which utilize an experienced and qualified interpreter. Rather, we add a qualitative perspective to an area that has been dominated by quantitative research to explore some of the linguistic dynamics of a consultation where all parties are to some degree bilingual.

9.3 Triadic medical consultations

Like Vickers *et al.* (2015), the consultation we are examining in this paper is triadic, and the addition of a family member to the doctor–patient dyad can alter the interactional dynamic. Vickers and colleagues note that in their wider corpus of consultations, those where the patient attended alone unfolded unproblematically in Spanish. It was only when a third party (a husband in one case, a daughter in another) was present that English entered the dialogue and the patient experienced disempowerment.

The dynamics of triadic consultations have received growing research interest within the fields of paediatrics and geriatrics in recent years (Adelman *et al.* 1987; Beisecker 1989; Coupland and Coupland 2000; see also Tates and Meeuwesen 2001 for an overview). It is now widely recognized that family members may play a variety of roles in the consultation, some of which are helpful while others undermine clear communication or patient agency. For example, Adelman *et al.* (1987) identified three stances family members or companions may take: the patient advocate, who is an activist for or extender of the patient, or a mediator for both doctor and patient; the passive observer who is disengaged from the exchange; or the antagonist who undermines the patient or acts opportunistically. Beisecker (1989) is an example of an early study that takes a very negative view of triadic consultations, seeing the companion as challenging and undermining the patient's own account and leading to the patient being discussed in the third person between the doctor and the companion (Beiscker 1989: 65). This is a recurrent theme in later studies (Risteen

Hasselkus 1994: 291; Tsai 2007; Vickers *et al.* 2015) and shows the linguistic challenges inherent in even monolingual triadic consultations.

The characterization of companions as always playing a negative role is too simplistic. Street and Gordon (2008) argue that the companion's involvement is often that of a watchdog or affected stakeholder who monitors the interaction and interjects questions, opinions and concerns when they feel certain issues need to be addressed (Street and Gordon 2008: 249). Family members have been shown to play a 'vital [role] in the development of the medical exchange' (Cordella 2011b: 348) by co-constructing the patient's account (Gordon *et al.* 2006; Lienard *et al.* 2008; Cordella 2011b). Two of the most common ways this was achieved in Cordella's studies of cancer medical consultations (Cordella 2011a, 2011b; Cordella and Poiani 2014) was by playing the role either of 'health advisor' who monitors and detects changes in the patient's health or of 'carer' who keeps track of the patient's health and well-being.

In our own work on interpreted medical consultations with older Italian Australians (Willoughby *et al.* 2015) we have found that talk between the doctor and accompanying family member may occur in English and not be interpreted into Italian, excluding and marginalizing the patient (see also Roberts and Sarangi, this volume). Family members' comments in Italian were also not consistently translated into English, undermining their ability to advocate for or support the patient. We thus wondered whether having a language-concordant doctor would ameliorate some of these issues, or whether the presence of a bilingual family member would undermine the language concordance of the consultation.

9.4 Data and methodology

In this paper we present data from one consultation recorded as part of a wider project investigating interpreted medical consultations for older Italian speakers in Melbourne, Australia (see Willoughby *et al.* 2015). For this consultation an interpreter had been booked but was cancelled when it became apparent that the doctor was a fluent Italian speaker. We had already negotiated consent to record the consultation from all parties, so decided to go ahead with the recording.

The recording took place at an outpatients' neurology clinic at a public hospital in the suburbs of Melbourne. Greater Melbourne has a large Italian-speaking population (as of 2016 some 101,000 individuals or 2.3%

of the city's population – idCommunity n.d.), mostly made up of post-war migrants and their descendants. The population of first-language (L1) Italian speakers (many of who speak dialects quite different from standard Italian) is now aging (Willoughby *et al.* 2015). However, there remains a significant number of 1.5- and second-generation speakers of Italian who are also fluent speakers of English – including the doctor and family member in this consultation.

The patient, who we shall call Anna, was attending the clinic for assessment of the effect of medication intended to improve her mobility. Anna is 70+ and a long-term resident of Australia. She is accompanied by her daughter, who is 40+ and works in health care. We are aware that the participants have different relations with the Italian language (Anna was born in Italy and speaks a regional variety of Italian, while her daughter and the doctor are members of the Italian-Australian speech community, but with different home varieties) but, within the interaction we analyse here, we see little if any evidence of intra-Italian variation and no miscommunication was perceived.

After all parties had given consent for the recording, each participant was provided with an individual radio microphone. The entire consultation was recorded on equipment in a room adjacent to the consultation room as three individual mono tracks, as well as a stereo mix. Although the stereo mix was the primary source for transcription, the individual tracks were referred to frequently, to clarify overlapping speech segments and to pick up back-channelling and self-directed speech. Transcriptions were done using the Du Bois system (Du Bois *et al.* 1993), as outlined in the Appendix, and include the verbatim transcription of non-standard language forms. Initial transcription was undertaken by either a fluent bilingual, who is also an accredited interpreter,[3] or a competent second-language speaker of Italian. Transcriptions and translations of Italian were checked by a second bilingual speaker.

We draw on broad discourse analysis methodologies to analyse and interpret one naturally occurring event. Our primary concern in the data analysis was identifying and accounting for recurrent patterns, with a focus on the local organization of talk and negotiation of meaning. As such, we are not simply presenting a case study of a typical consultation, but rather what Mitchell (1984) terms a 'telling case'; that is, a close analysis which allows the analyst to tease out the theoretical aspects of an event or situation. As our consultation turned out to unfold quite smoothly, a concern was to identify the patterns of interaction which instantiate good communication and the factors which facilitate that.

9.5 Analysis

In the following section we analyse the main themes in the medical consultation.

The dominant language frame

As will become clear, an important feature of this consultation is that Italian is spoken almost exclusively by all parties, and this ensures that the patient is included in all aspects of the consultation. The opening sequence of the consultation (Extract 1) illustrates this strong Italian frame, with the doctor immediately beginning in Italian and addressing the patient directly.

Excerpt 1: Consultation opening (D = doctor; FM = family member; P = patient)

[door closed]
1 D: Allora come va?
so how are you?
2 P: (Hx) non c'è male
(Hx) not too bad
3 D: e :::
and:::
4 da quando ti ha smesso quel Motilium è diventata
since you stopped taking that Motilium
5 p-più meglio con movimento
has your movement improved
6 P: Sì
Yes

The transcript of the interaction consists of 2062 word tokens (as counted by MS Word). Seventeen of these are names of drugs, people or places where language choice is not relevant. Of the remaining 2045 word tokens, 160 are English. This count includes 26 tokens of *yeah*, 20 of *ok* and 5 tokens of *alright*. English tokens make up just under 8% of the total, but if the assent tokens are ignored this figure drops to 5%.

We noted in the methodology section that the doctor, patient and family member all speak different varieties of Italian and bring different proficiencies in English to the consultation. As Extract 1 illustrates, the doctor and patient understand each other's Italian easily, and we will later see that this is true for the family member as well. Indeed, a striking feature of this consultation is that we can identify no obvious instances of miscommunication in the consultation. We believe three features that promote strong understanding in this consultation are the commitment by all parties to using Italian, the doctor's strong fluency in Italian and the proactive role the family member takes in supporting and occasionally correcting her mother's account of affairs.

The family member's role

In this consultation, the daughter plays a vital 'health advisor' (Cordella 2011a, 2011b) role in supporting, adding to and occasionally contradicting the patient's account of affairs. When medical consultations are interpreted, bilingual family members may have to make strategic choices about what language to use in playing this role. Their comments in Italian may not be interpreted, while their comments in English might exclude the patient and encourage the tendency of doctors and family members to address each other rather than the patient, as has been noted for geriatric encounters (Risteen Hasselkus 1994: 304). This problem disappears when all parties in the consultation share some fluency in a common language and are committed to using that language in the interaction. In Extract 2, for example, we see the daughter reinforcing her mother's statements about how her mobility has improved under a new treatment regime.

Excerpt 2

1 D: E quando che va a letto (..) può andare
and when you go to bed (..) can you go
2 a letto (.) può girarsi (.)
to bed can you turn over
3 può escere dal letto/
can you get out of bed/
4 P: sì sì (1) sì posso fare (.)
yes yes I can do that
5 Beh (.) non ho disturbo (.) no
no I don't have any problems no
6 D: Ok
7 P: Devo scendere piano piano dal letto
I have to get out of bed very slowly
8 (H) prima n::: (1.5) non potevo
(H) before (1.5) I wasn't able
9 scendere dal letto
to get out of bed

10 FM: Prima non non si non si poteva
before she couldn't couldn't
11 nemmeno girare nel letto
even turn over in bed
12 D: mm (..) ok

Here the daughter's comments serve several related purposes that could not all be achieved if the doctor and patient did not share the same language. The daughter's contribution demonstrates that Anna's previous assessment of her mobility was not hyperbolic – before the new treatment she really could not turn over in bed and now there has been a dramatic improvement. The daughter's assessment also aligns to the patient's description, adding to the collaborative and affiliative discourse achieved by the use of the patient's preferred language.

The daughter also plays an important role in reinforcing the patient's comments by providing more information at points where she feels her mother has been unclear or not as informative as required, as in Extract 3.

Excerpt 3

1 D: ma è indipendente può fare tutto se stessa
but you're independent you can do everything by yourself
2 non le occorre aiuto
you don't need help
3 P: sì sì sì
yes yes yes
4 D: [inaudible]
5 FM: sì sì no fa tutto se stessa
yes yes no she does everything herself
6 solo c'ha il comune che viene
except that she has the council come
7 a pulire ogni seconda settimana
to clean every second week

On this occasion, the daughter's comment gives added strength to the general message that her mother is independent and can manage most everyday tasks for herself. It does however qualify the patient's previous assessment by making the doctor aware that she receives help for more physically demanding cleaning tasks such as vacuuming. Such discourse illustrates the daughter's high level of health literacy and reminds us that an ability to understand the direction of the doctor's questioning is a key component of ensuring smooth communication in this consultation.

The clearest example of the family member pre-empting miscommunication in this exchange is given in Extract 4, where the daughter explicitly contradicts an incorrect statement made by the patient.

Excerpt 4

1 D: ma c'ha disturbo con la vista Lei/ (2) no/
but you have problems with your eyesight no/
2 P: no non c'è disturbo con la vista\
no I don't have problems with my eyesight
3 D: cosa (.) non c'ha cataract/ a::: (.)glaucoma
what (.) no cataracts? a:::
4 (1) oh (..) so (.) ok (.) ok (..)
5 yeah what (.) no c'ha cataract/ a:::
you don't have cataract/
6 FM: actually she does have cataracts (.)
7 yeah and she's got glaucoma as well yeah
8 So she's taking um she's she's yeah yeah
9 c'ha prende la medicina per glaucoma
she's taking medicine for glaucoma
10 per la pressione
for the pressure
11 pressure in the eyes

In response to the doctor's question about her eyesight, Anna provides a negative statement 'no no there isn't any problem with my sight'. Nevertheless, the doctor persists, moving from Italian to English, adding 'no cataracts er glaucoma' (line 3). This is answered by the patient's daughter using a pre-disclosure of information token (*actually*), which shows that the information to be disclosed differs from that given by the patient. In her refutation of the patient's claim the daughter has codeswitched to English, possibly to soften the face threat implied by her utterance, or perhaps because of her haste to ensure that this misinformation is corrected, or because the doctor's use of English may have provided a trigger. This statement is followed by a number of false starts in English before she moves back into an Italian frame to complete the statement that the patient is taking medicine to control the pressure in her eyes. The daughter's short incursion into English is quickly self-corrected, ensuring that her mother remains aware of what is being said and can correct her daughter's account should she feel the need to do so.

Drawing on English

The data above suggest that the case study is a largely monolingual triadic consultation, but the bilingual competence of the participants contributes to effective communication.

While the consultation has a strongly Italian frame, both the doctor and the family member occasionally use English medical terms, generally in contexts where it appears they do not know (or at least cannot recall) an Italian equivalent. Extract 5 is an example of this.

Excerpt 5

1 D: cos'è specialista [chirurgo chirurgo oh sk-
what's he specialist surgeon surgeon oh sk-
2 **dermatologist**
3 FM: specialista skin specialist (.) m:::
specialist skin specialist (.) mm
4 (..) dermatologist

In this extract the doctor's repetition of *chirurgo* suggests he is having difficulty recalling the Italian title for this type of specialist. He then switches to English with a change of state token *oh* and half-articulates *sk-*, which seems likely to be the English word *skin*, immediately amended to *dermatologist.* In the ensuing discourse the daughter also appears to search for an Italian equivalent, beginning with *specialista*, before continuing in English with *skin specialist* and then, after further hesitation (and possible word search in Italian), taking up the doctor's term *dermatologist*.

An example of the bias towards English for the introduction of medical terminology occurs in Extract 4 above. The term *glaucoma* is used there; this term is orthographically identical in English and Italian, but the pronunciation is different, particularly in the vowel of the first syllable. In the relevant exchange, the doctor produced one token of the word in an Italian frame (although he has code-switched for *cataracts* a few words earlier) and the family member produces two tokens, one in an English frame and one in an Italian frame. But all three tokens have (Australian) English pronunciation; the first vowel is [o:] or [ɔ] and not [au] as it would be in Italian.

In Vickers *et al.* (2015), the analysis assumes that the Spanish-speaking patients attending the clinic do not understand any English. In our study, all the older Italian-speaking patients understood at least simple English, unsurprising given that they had lived in Australia for most of their adult lives. Interpreters and bilingual doctors were utilized because Italian was the language in which the patients felt most comfortable discussing complex medical issues, not because they necessarily had very low English proficiency. This creates a somewhat different dynamic to the study by Vickers and colleagues: on the one hand the use of some simple English need not be exclusionary, but on the other hand judging when the patient has reached the limit of their English abilities can be difficult and potentially face-threatening – particularly if the patient persists in trying to say in English something that they are having difficulty expressing (Willoughby *et al.* 2015).

In this consultation, the patient produces only seven English tokens and all of these are single words or idioms embedded in complete utterances in Italian, as shown in Extract 6.

Excerpt 6

(a) le immagino sempre e mi faccio **upset**
*I imagine them all the time and it makes me **upset***

(b) perche' adesso adesso l'abbiamo l'abbiamo (.) ***discovered*** ma (..) io ce l'avevo da prima
*because now now we have we have (.) **discovered** it but (..) I had it before*

(c) pensavano che aveva avuto un **stroke**
*they thought that I had had a **stroke***

(d) certe volte mi fa perdere il bilancio quando non sono **steady** di camminare
*sometimes it makes me lose my balance when I am not **steady** to walk*

(e) beh (.) fà un pochino **up and down** insomma
well (.) it goes up and down a bit overall

Of these, example (b) suggests the patient not being able to remember an Italian word; the English token is preceded by false starts and a hesitation. The other four cases are all fluent uses of English tokens in the Italian matrix. Strikingly, all these English words are used for negative experiences of the patient.

While the doctor normally consults in English, he accommodates to the patient's clear preference for Italian and always addresses her directly in that language. The daughter is not quite so rigid in adhering to the Italian frame of the consultation, sometimes addressing both her mother and the doctor in English. Often these beginnings in English are self-corrected, as in Extract 4 above and Extract 7 below.

Excerpt 7

1 FM: I'll just tell him about that other condition
2 that you have um I don't know if I've told you
3 (1) se l'abbiamo detto che (6) (Hx) um:::
If I told you that (6) (Hx) um
4 (1) non so se se l'ho detto l'altra volta
(1) *I don't know if I told you the other time*
5 che lei c'ha anche (H) ah
That she also has (H) ah
6 lipodermatoschlerosis nelle gambe
lipodermatoschlerosis in her legs
7 (1.5) che gli da' tanto disturbo
(1.5) that makes her very uncomfortable

By repeating in Italian what she initially said in English to the doctor, and then continuing in Italian as she explained medical information, the daughter shows strong awareness of her mother's language preference and her own willingness to engage in Italian. This move back to Italian for medical discussion not only ensures the patient is fully included in the conversation but helps preserve the strong Italian frame of the consultation, with utterances in English treated as marked deviations that should be corrected. Not all such utterances are corrected, however, with Extract 8 providing one of the few examples in this consultation of the doctor producing extended discourse in English.

Excerpt 8

1 FM: I notice she has more swing in her arm/
2 than she did [before/ (.) m:::]
3 D: [yeah yeah (..)] the left one isn't as good but
4 FM: yeah yeah cos that's the left
5 is always the weakest (1.5) m:::m:::
6 P: questo qua è quello che non è buono
this one here is the one that's not good
7 le braccia la gamba
the arms the leg

At this point, the patient had been asked to stand up and walk around so that the doctor could assess the effect of treatment on her mobility. The patient was thus physically distant from the others during this exchange, which is perhaps best viewed as an evaluative aside. However, this does not exclude the patient from the discourse; on the contrary, she seems to understand what has been said and chimes in at the end with a comment in Italian that reinforces the doctor's and the daughter's assessment. We thus might view this exchange as a case of the patient acknowledging and accommodating to the language preference of her daughter, and as evidence that the use of some English is not automatically exclusionary.

9.6 Discussion

From this analysis, several clear points of contrast emerge with the consultations discussed by Vickers and colleagues and may account for the fact that our consultation appeared to proceed very smoothly and include the patient, whereas theirs contained many moments where the patient was excluded or disempowered. One of the simplest points is that all parties were clearly committed to using Italian as the default language of the consultation, and extended discourse in English was almost always repaired. This seems to be something of a rarity in consultations involving family members where – regardless of whether a family member or professional interpreter is in attendance – long asides between the doctor and family members in English are often not translated for the patient (see e.g. Willoughby *et al.* 2015, Roberts and Sarangi, this volume). The roles played by the accompanying family members in our study and the Vickers study are also quite different. The literature on monolingual triadic consultations has already made clear that some family members play important roles in ensuring the patient receives the best possible care, while others interrupt and undermine the patient's contribution (cf. Beisecker 1989; Cordella 2011b; Sarangi, this volume). Our work and that of Vickers and colleagues shows that this contrast also exists in bilingual triadic consultations. The positive or negative contribution of the family member is arguably amplified in the bilingual context, since the opportunity to exclude the patient from the discourse is even greater if the doctor and the companion converse about the patient in a language that the patient does not understand well.

Similar comments can be made in comparing this consultation with those we have previously described which included an interpreter (Willoughby *et al.* 2015). The current data illustrate a preference from all parties to interact in their best common language, Italian. We have shown a similar preference in our previous study, but the common language there is English and the capacities of the parties to use that language vary. The interpreter is there to assist when English fails, but this brings problems as noted by Vickers *et al.* (2015: 156):

> Interpretation is of course a kind of code-switching that takes place in the medical consultation, and as studies of interpretation demonstrate, it is the person who has access to both languages in use in the medical consultation who carries the interactional power.

Our previous study showed that these problems arose particularly in regard to accompanying family members. The interpreter has to make decisions about the extent to which the contributions of that interactant are relevant and need interpreting, and we noted that such decisions do impact the completeness of communication. We certainly would not argue that issues of interactional power are not relevant to the discourse we have examined here, but we do suggest that the commitment of all parties to use the patient's preferred language means that at least some of those issues are minimized.

9.7 Conclusions

In this consultation, communication between the doctor, the patient and the family member is smooth and a clear Italian frame is maintained throughout. Access to a bilingual doctor ensures direct communication between the patient and the doctor and that the family member's comments appear on record. Despite being fluent English speakers, the doctor and the family member make a concerted effort to speak Italian throughout the consultation, and this is key for including the patient. English continues to play a role in medical terminology and is used by the daughter to introduce complex or disaffiliative information (i.e. as discussed in Extract 4 with the pre-disclosure marker '*actually*')

Another factor that has likely influenced the clear communication in this consultation is the supportive and proactive health advisor role taken by the family member. We have illustrated the many small supportive moves the daughter makes in this consultation to support and extend her mother's contributions and occasionally to correct or clarify information. Importantly too, the daughter plays this health advisor role without taking over the conversation and shifting it to a discussion primarily between herself and the physician, as is often the case in geriatric triadic medical encounters (Risteen Hasselkus 1994). The fact that all parties share a common language is key to this communicative success and is an area where bilingual doctors have a clear advantage in managing the contribution of family members over monolingual doctors working with interpreters.

This might suggest that bilingual doctors should be encouraged to conduct medical consultations in the primary language of their patients, since this may increase patients' participation (see also Fernandez *et al.* 2004; Green *et al.* 2005) and decrease miscommunication. While this option would bring some benefits to the medical consultations, contrasting our results with Vickers *et al.* (2015) shows that bilingual consultations are not a panacea. Because patients and the companions are rarely totally monolingual, bilingual health care workers may find themselves having to negotiate language choice in a complex way in consultations. This may prove particularly challenging in consultations with more controlling companions and is an area where bilingual health care workers may benefit from training before they begin practising in a minority language. Given that many doctors in the US and Australia are already practising in the languages of their patients, rather than in English, there is also a pressing need for more research in this area in order to better understand the mechanics of how such consultations unfold. Such research must explore how factors such as the doctor's, the patient's and accompanying family members' proficiencies in both the minority language and in English affect the consultation, as well as if and how doctors negotiate intercultural differences in the health beliefs or expected consulting style of their migrant-background patients, compared to patients from the wider society (see also Sarangi, this volume).

In conclusion, it is very important to note that the doctor in this consultation is a fluent Italian speaker working in a context where an interpreter would be provided at no cost to either the patient or the hospital if he chose not to consult in Italian. This context means the doctor is not under systemic pressure to practice in Italian and likely has the effect that only practitioners who are truly fluent and comfortable consulting in a language other than English elect to do so. This stands in contrast to reports from the US of doctors who are imperfect second-language learners consulting in Spanish (Yoon *et al.* 2004; Green *et al.* 2005), and stands as a reminder that bilingual doctors are best seen as complementing, not replacing, a health system that provides professional interpreters in medical consultations.

Appendix: Transcription symbols

Unit	Truncated syllable (first)	,
	Truncated syllable (middle and final)	-
Speakers	Speaker identity/turn start	:
	Overlapping talk begins	[
	Overlapping talk ends	]
Tone	Low falling tone	\
	Rising tone	/
Pause/Silence	Silence timed in seconds	(1)
	Pause of less than half a second	(.)
	Pause longer than half a second)	(..)
Vocal Noises	Inhalation	(H)
	Exhalation	(Hx)
Quality voice	Emphasis	EMPHASIS
	Perceived change based on volume or pitch change	
Lengthening	Vowel/ consonant elongation	:::
Transcribers' perspective	Researcher's comment	(( ))
	Uncertain hearing	<X X>

Notes

1 In 2011 over half of Australia's GPs and 47% of specialists were born overseas (ABS 2014). A survey by Ryan *et al.* (2016) of 146 final year medical students at an Australian university found that 73% spoke a language other than English at home (Ryan *et al.* 2016: 140), reinforcing the idea that the Australian medical workforce is highly multilingual.

2 Ryan *et al.* (2019: 140) explicitly asked whether any of the medical students in their sample held interpreting qualifications; none did so.

3 Accredited by the Australian National Accreditation Authority for Interpreters and Translators (NAATI).

References

Adelman, Ronald D., Michele G. Greene and Rita Charon (1987) The physician–elderly patient–companion triad in the medical encounter: The development of a conceptual framework and research agenda. *Gerontologist* 27 (6): 729–734. https://doi.org/10.1093/geront/27.6.729

Australian Bureau of Statistics (2013) *Doctors and Nurses*. Australian Social Trends April 2013. Online: https://www.abs.gov.au/AUSSTATS/abs@.nsf/Lookup/4102.0Main+Features20April+2013

Baker, David W., Risa Hayes and Julia P. Fortier (1998) Interpreter use and satisfaction with interpersonal aspects of care for Spanish-speaking patients. *Medical Care* 36 (10): 1461–1470. https://doi.org/10.1097/00005650-199810000-00004

Beisecker, Analee E. (1989) The influence of a companion on the doctor-elderly patient interaction. *Health Communication* 1 (1): 55–70. https://doi.org/10.1207/s15327027hc0101_7

Britt, Helena, Graeme C. Miller, Clare Bayram, Joan Henderson, Lisa Valenti, Christopher Harrison, Ying Pan *et al.* (2016) A Decade of Australian General Practice Activity 2006–07 to 2015–16. Sydney: Sydney University Press.

Chao, Maria T., Margaret A. Handley, Judy Quan, Urmimala Sarkar, Neda Ratanawongsa and Dean Schillinger (2015) Disclosure of complementary health approaches among low income and racially diverse safety net patients with diabetes. *Patient Education and Counseling* 98 (11): 1360-1366. https://doi.org/10.1016/j.pec.2015.06.011

Cordella, Marisa (2011a) Enfrentándose al cáncer en compañía: el rol del familiar en la consulta. *Discurso & Sociedad* 5 (3): 469–491.

Cordella, Marisa (2011b) A triangle that may work well: Looking through the angles of a three-way exchange in cancer medical encounters. *Discourse & Communication* 5 (4): 337–353. https://doi.org/10.1177/1750481311418100

Cordella, Marisa and Aldo Poiani (2014) *Behavioural Oncology: Psychological, Communicative and Social Dimensions.* New York: Springer. https://doi.org/10.1007/978-1-4614-9605-2

Coupland, Nikolas and Justine Coupland (2000) Relational frames and pronominal address/reference: The discourse of geriatric medical triads. In Srikant Sarangi and Malcolm Coulthard (eds) *Discourse and Social Life*, 207–229. London: Pearson.

Du Bois, John W. S., Stephan Schuetze-Coburn, Susanna Cumming and Danae Paolino (1993) Outline of discourse transcription. In Jane A. Edwards and Martin D. Lampert (eds) *Talking Data: Transcription and Coding in Discourse Research*, 45–89. Hillsdale, NJ: Lawrence Erlbaum Associates.

Dunlap, Jonathan L., Joshua D. Jaramillo, Raji Koppolu, Robert Wright, Fernando Mendoza and Matias Bruzoni (2015) The effects of language concordant care on patient satisfaction and clinical understanding for Hispanic pediatric surgery patients. *Journal of Pediatric Surgery* 50 (9): 1586–1589. https://doi.org/10.1016/j.jpedsurg.2014.12.020

Fernandez, Alicia, Dean Schillinger, Kevin Grumbach, Anne Rosenthal, Anita L. Stewart, Frances Wang and Eliseo J. Pérez-Stable (2004) Physician language ability and cultural competence. *Journal of General Internal Medicine* 19 (2): 167–174. https://doi.org/10.1111/j.1525-1497.2004.30266.x

Gordon, Howard S., Richard L. Street Jr., Barbara F. Sharf and Julianne Souchek (2006) Racial differences in doctors' information-giving and patients' participation. *Cancer* 107 (6): 1313–1320. https://doi.org/10.1002/cncr.22122

Green, Alexander, Quyen Ngo-Metzger, Anna T. R. Legedza, Michael P. Massagli, Russell S. Phillips and Lisa I. Iezzoni (2005) Interpreter services, language concordance, and health care quality. *Journal of General Internal Medicine* 20 (11): 1050–1056. https://doi.org/10.1111/j.1525-1497.2005.0223.x

Hampers, Louis C. and Jennifer E. McNulty (2002) Professional interpreters and bilingual physicians in a pediatric emergency department: Effect on resource utilization. *Archives of Pediatrics & Adolescent Medicine* 156 (11): 1108–1113. https://doi.org/10.1001/archpedi.156.11.1108

idCommunity (n.d.) Greater Melbourne: Language spoken at home. Available online: https://profile.id.com.au/australia/language?WebID=260

Lee, Linda J., Holly A. Batal, Judith H. Maselli and Jean S. Kutner (2002) Effect of Spanish interpretation method on patient satisfaction in an urban walk-in clinic. *Journal of General Internal Medicine* 17 (8): 641–646. https://doi.org/10.1046/j.1525-1497.2002.10742.x

Lienard, Aurore, Isabelle Merckaert, Yves Libert, Nicole Delvaux, Serge Marchal, Jacques Boniver, Anne-Marie Etienne *et al.* (2008) Factors that influence cancer patients' and relatives' anxiety following a three-person medical consultation: Impact of a communication skills training program for physicians. *Psycho-Oncology* 17 (5): 488–496. https://doi.org/10.1002/pon.1262

Masland, Mary C., Soo H. Kang and Yifei Ma (2011) Association between limited English proficiency and understanding prescription labels among five ethnic groups in California. *Ethnicity & Health* 16 (2): 125–144. https://doi.org/10.1080/13557858.2010.543950

Mitchell, J. Clyde (1984). Typicality and the case study. In Roy F. Ellen (ed.) *Ethnographic Research: A Guide to General Conduct*, 237–241. London: Academic Press.

Ngo-Metzger, Quyen, Dara H. Sorkin, Russell S. Phillips, Sheldon Greenfield, Michael P. Massagli, Brian Clarridge and Sherrie H. Kaplan (2007) Providing high-quality care for limited English proficient patients: The importance of language concordance and interpreter use. *Journal of General Internal Medicine* 22 (suppl. 2): 324–330. https://doi.org/10.1007/s11606-007-0340-z

O'Brien, Matthew and Judy Shea (2011) Disparities in patient satisfaction among Hispanics: The role of language preference. *Journal of Immigrant and Minority Health / Center for Minority Public Health* 13 (2): 408–412. https://doi.org/10.1007/s10903-009-9275-2

Risteen Hasselkus, Betty (1994) Three-track care: Older patient, family member, and physician in the medical visit. *Journal of Aging Studies* 8 (3): 291–307. https://doi.org/10.1016/0890-4065(94)90005-1

Ryan, Anna T., Caleb Fisher and Neville Chiavaroli (2019) Medical students as interpreters in health care situations: '... It's a grey area'. *Medical Journal of Australia* 211 (4): 170–174. https://doi.org/10.5694/mja2.50235

Street, Richard L. and Howard S. Gordon (2008) Companion participation in cancer consultations. *Psycho-Oncology* 17 (3): 244–251. https://doi.org/10.1002/pon.1225

Sudore, Rebecca L., C. Seth Landefeld, Eliseo J. Pérez-Stable, Kirsten Bibbins-Doming, Brie A. Williams and Dean Schillinger (2009) Unraveling the relationship between literacy, language proficiency, and patient–physician communication. *Patient Education and Counseling* 75 (3): 398–402. https://doi.org/10.1016/j.pec.2009.02.019

Tates, Kiek and Ludwien Meeuwesen (2001) Doctor–parent–child communication: A (re)view of the literature. *Social Science & Medicine* 52 (6): 839–851. https://doi.org/10.1016/S0277-9536(00)00193-3

Tsai, Mei-hui (2007) Who gets to talk? An alternative framework evaluating companion effects in geriatric triads. *Communication & Medicine* 4 (1): 37–49. https://doi.org/10.1515/CAM.2007.005

Vertovec, Steven (2007) Super-diversity and its implications. *Ethnic and Racial Studies* 30 (6): 1024–1054. https://doi.org/10.1080/01419870701599465

Vickers, Caroline H., Ryan Goble and Sharon K. Deckert (2015) Third party interaction in the medical context: Code-switching and control. *Journal of Pragmatics* 84: 154–171. https://doi.org/10.1016/j.pragma.2015.05.009

Willoughby, Louisa, Simon Musgrave, Marisa Cordella and Julie Bradshaw (2015) Being heard: The role of family members in bilingual medical consultations. In Elke Stracke (ed.) *Intersections: Applied Linguistics as a Meeting Place*, 22–42. Newcastle upon Tyne, UK: Cambridge Scholars Publishing.

Wilson, Elisabeth, Alice Hm Chen, Kevin Grumbach, Frances Wang and Alicia Fernandez (2005) Effects of limited English proficiency and physician language on health care comprehension. *Journal of General Internal Medicine* 20 (9): 800–806. https://doi.org/10.1111/j.1525-1497.2005.0174.x

Yoon, Jean, Kevin Grumbach and Andrew B. Bindman (2004) Access to Spanish-speaking physicians in California: Supply, insurance, or both. *Journal of the American Board of Family Practice* 17 (3): 165–72. https://doi.org/10.3122/jabfm.17.3.165

Louisa Willoughby, PhD, is a Associate Professor in the Linguistics Program at Monash University. Her research focuses on issues affecting speakers of minority languages, particularly in education and health settings. She is also interested in language maintenance and shift more broadly, language and identity and Deaf studies. Address for correspondence: School of Languages, Literatures, Cultures and Linguistics, Faculty of Arts, 20 Chancellors Walk Monash University Vic Australia 3800.
Email: Louisa.Willoughby@monash.edu

Marisa Cordella holds a PhD in linguistics from Monash University and is currently a Reader in Spanish at the University of Queensland. Her research interests include discourse analysis, intercultural communication, medical discourse, translation studies and intergenerational second-language learning. Address for correspondence: School of Languages & Comparative Cultural Studies, University of Queensland, Qld, Australia 4072.
Email: m.cordella@uq.edu.au

Simon Musgrave, PhD, is an Adjunct Research Fellow in the Linguistics Program at Monash University and Engagement Lead for the Language Data Commons of Australia project. His research interests include Austronesian languages, language endangerment, African languages in Australia, communication in medical encounters and linguistics as part of digital humanities. Address for correspondence: School of Languages, Literatures, Cultures and Linguistics, Faculty of Arts, 20 Chancellors Walk Monash University Vic Australia 3800. Email: Simon.Musgrave@monash.edu

Julie Bradshaw has a PhD from the University of York, UK, and is an Adjunct Research Fellow in the Linguistics Program at Monash University. Her

research interests include multilingualism and language maintenance, the sociolinguistic aspects of second-language acquisition, minority-language literacy, place-identity and communication in medical settings. Address for correspondence: School of Languages, Literatures, Cultures and Linguistics, Faculty of Arts, 20 Chancellors Walk Monash University Vic Australia 3800.
Email: Julie.Bradshaw@monash.edu

10 Interpreter-mediated aphasia assessments: Mismatches in frames and professional orientations

Peter Roger & Chris Code

10.1 Introduction

Speech pathologists (also known as speech-language pathologists or speech therapists) are professionals with expertise in the assessment and management of a range of communication disorders, both developmental and acquired. One of the commonest conditions encountered in the speech pathology clinic is *aphasia*, which is defined by the second edition of the Boston Diagnostic Aphasia Examination (BDAE-2) as 'the disturbance of any or all of the skills, associations and habits of spoken or written language produced by injury to certain brain areas that are specialized for these functions' (Goodglass and Kaplan 1983: 5). The most common cause of aphasia is a cerebrovascular accident (or 'stroke'), and following such an event, a speech pathologist is commonly called upon to provide an assessment of the person's communicative abilities. Where the patient and the speech pathologist do not share the same language, either a bilingual aide (who may be a family member, or an informal 'interpreter' that the health service can access) or a professional interpreter is generally called upon to assist with the assessment and subsequent therapy program.

In Australia, the professional association representing speech pathologists advises its members that professional accredited interpreters must be engaged in such situations whenever possible (Speech Pathology Australia n.d.). Some state government healthcare policies also mandate that individuals should have access to interpreters when necessary

(Siyambalapitiya and Davidson 2015), and parts of the country have well-established healthcare interpreter services that coordinate the supply of interpreters for the public health system. The National Accreditation Authority for Translators and Interpreters (NAATI) certifies professional interpreters to practice in healthcare settings at various levels and for a variety of languages. Roger *et al.* (2000) found that more than 95% of speech pathologists surveyed across metropolitan Sydney reported using interpreters when assessing and treating people with aphasia when the person's first language was not English. Many of those responding to the survey also reported that they found the assessment of aphasia through an interpreter particularly difficult, and were often less than satisfied with the way that such sessions unfolded.

Although a number of very useful recommendations have been put forward for speech pathologists and interpreters working collaboratively, there have been few studies which look at the discourse of such clinical encounters in order to identify the precise moments at which difficulties manifest. The aim of the present study is to identify and describe in detail these 'critical moments' when the two professionals involved appear to have divergent understandings of the goals or purposes associated with their interaction. A detailed understanding of such moments could feed into professional development and training for speech pathologists and interpreters.

The following section reviews the literature on interpreter-mediated assessment of aphasia and provides an overview of interactive framing, with a particular focus on its application in studies of healthcare interactions. The methodology employed in this study is then outlined, and the findings are presented with illustrative extracts from two of the five recorded aphasia assessments. These findings are discussed in the context of the literature, and the paper concludes with recommendations for ways in which the contribution of interpreters to aphasia assessments could be more effectively managed.

10.2 Literature review

Interpreters in the assessment of aphasia

There is a growing recognition within professional bodies representing both speech pathology and community interpreting of the unique challenges that arise in interpreter-mediated language assessments. From an interpreting perspective, Frey *et al.* (1990) point out that interpreters in speech pathology settings often work outside the normal interpreting role, becoming more an 'assistant' to the speech pathologist than a professional interpreter. They argue that this can be justified on the grounds that it permits equality of access by members of minority language groups to speech pathology services, although they also recommend that interpreters' consent be sought prior to asking them to act in this capacity. Gentile *et al.* (1996) also discuss interpreting in the speech pathology context, but argue that it does not involve a re-definition of the interpreter's role:

> The demands on the interpreter are in many ways similar to those in mental health: to render into the other language what can be rendered, and to accurately describe what can't. [...] It is important that the interpreter not misunderstand their role. In describing the subject's speech, they are not being asked to change professional roles with the speech therapist. (Gentile *et al.* 1996: 26)

The expectation that interpreters provide 'descriptions' of the speech of individuals with aphasia can be a cause for concern among some interpreters, who feel that they might be asked to give what amounts to an 'opinion' on an aspect of language that was outside their sphere of expertise (Clark 1998).

From the speech pathology perspective, Whitworth and Sjardin highlight the need for specific training of interpreters 'in the complexities of the assessment process' (Whitworth and Sjardin 1993: 134). It follows that any need for specific training would apply equally to speech pathologists. Isaac (2002) sets out in detail a 'collaborative partnership' model for speech pathologists and interpreters working together, and stresses the importance of mutual understanding and professional respect.

An encounter which involves a speech pathologist and an interpreter brings together two 'language professionals'. It would seem at first glance that this shared element underpinning the two professions, and the fact that they are operating in a healthcare context, should help them to work together. In this respect, they are members of a common 'community of interest', a term coined by Sarangi (2015: 29) to describe 'scenarios in which one crosses different communities of discourse/interpretive practice – where one may share "interests" but not "practices", "discourses" and "interpretations"'. A crucial issue here is the way in which 'language' is conceptualized as part of the *knowledge schema* – defined by

Tannen and Wallat (1993: 60) as 'participants' expectations about people, objects, events and setting is the world' – typically associated with each profession.

Broadly speaking, the interpreter's professional work centres around *meaning*; central to their role is the need to convey accurately and completely to both parties what has been said in an encounter (National Accreditation Authority for Translators and Interpreters 2000). Where a speaker's intended meaning is unclear or ambiguous, it follows that community interpreters must seek clarification in order to enable them to perform their role. In contrast, the speech pathologist's professional knowledge schema centres around ways in which 'normal' language and communication can be disrupted by acquired or developmental disorders. Many of the diagnostic assessments that they carry out may thus focus to a large extent on *form*. Specifically, they need to determine the extent to which a person with a communication disorder can understand normally formed language, as well as document the ways in which the language produced by this person deviates from what is considered 'normal' (at the levels of phonology, syntax, lexis, discourse and pragmatics). Speech pathologists thus expect to encounter frequent instances where an individual has difficulty understanding or expressing ideas, and their assessment procedures involve the identification of the details of such breakdowns before seeking to overcome them.

Merlini and Favaron (2005) provide a detailed analysis of aspects of the discourse of interpreter-mediated speech pathology sessions. They draw on a number of analytical techniques to illustrate the ways in which the two professionals working cooperatively allows them to approach the ideal of what has been described as 'humane medical care'. The present study also examines clinical settings involving speech pathologist, interpreter and person with aphasia, but focuses instead on providing a systematic analysis of the apparent difficulties that arise in the communication between the two professional parties in the course of the interaction.

Interactive framing in clinical encounters

The theoretical framework employed here is interactive framing. Goffman set out a comprehensive theory of framing in his book *Frame Analysis* (Goffman 1974), using the question 'what is it that's going on here?' as his point of departure. A central tenet of the concept of interactive framing is that one's perspective (explicitly or implicitly understood) on the particular frame in which a given activity is taking place will determine the way in which messages will be interpreted.

Studies that have used forms of frame analysis to examine interactions in clinical settings have most often focused on aspects of the exchanges between the health professional and patient/client. A variety of clinical settings have been the subject of research, including aged care (Coupland *et al.* 1994), audiology (Coupland and Jaworski 1997), gynaecology (Beck and Ragan 1992), medical doctor training (Thomassen 2009), paediatrics (Tannen and Wallat 1993) and psychiatry (Ribeiro 1993; Ribeiro and Bastos 2005). To our knowledge, however, frame analysis has not been previously used in interaction-based studies of encounters in speech pathology (with or without interpreters).

The present study draws specifically on the work of Tannen and Wallat (1993), who focus on the way in which mismatched knowledge schemata trigger frame shifts in an encounter involving a paediatrician, child and mother. It also employs elements of the model for discourse studies of interpreter-mediated interaction set out by Wadensjö (1998), including Goffman's concept of *participation framework,* which emphasizes the way in which participants in an interaction constantly evaluate and re-evaluate their roles as the interaction unfolds (see also Goodwin 1981, 2000). Elements of Goffman's participation framework have been operationalized by subsequent researchers focusing on interactions in a range of professional contexts. Halvorsen and Sarangi (2015), for instance, demonstrate how the concepts of 'activity role' and 'discourse role' help to advance our understanding of the fluidity of participants' roles in a team meeting context. Wadensjö's work is particularly useful in operationalizing the notion of 'footing' in interpreter-mediated interactions.

Goffman's concept of *production format* is explained as the positions (or footings) that an individual adopts while producing a particular utterance (Wadensjö 1998). In this model, an individual can act as *animator* (a mere mouthpiece giving sound to an utterance), *author* (responsible only for the assembly and synthesis of information and giving it 'form' by composing/scripting the actual 'lines') or *principal* (assuming complete responsibility for the utterance and the intentions and beliefs which gave rise to it).

To complement this production format, Wadensjö proposes analogous categories that relate to the way in which individuals can align themselves to the utterances of others – for this she uses the term *reception format.* Each of the three receptive modes invite the hearer to take on a particular production role in his or her subsequent utterances. Assuming or being given the role of *reporter* naturally leads to the adoption of the animator's stance. Assuming or being given the role of *recapitulator* indicates that one was expected to take up the roles of both animator and author. Finally, being assigned or taking the role of *responder* leads one to adopt the role of animator, author and principal in a subsequent utterance. Difficulties can arise in interpreter-mediated encounters when the interpreter is unsure which of these possible reception format roles is being invoked by the other parties present.

10.3 Method

The data for this study were gathered by video-recording actual interpreter-mediated aphasia assessments which had been scheduled by the speech pathologists concerned.

All speech pathologists were employed at the same rehabilitation hospital within the metropolitan Sydney region, and routinely assessed and provided therapy (with the assistance of interpreters) to individuals with aphasia from a wide range of language backgrounds. Research ethics approval was obtained at both the university and hospital. Approval was also sought from the director of the relevant Health Care Interpreter Service, which supplied interpreters for the purposes of the aphasia assessments.

Assessments were conducted in the office of the relevant speech pathologist. With the consent of all parties, a video camera was set up in the room prior to each assessment session, and the session was observed from an adjacent room through a one-way window. In order to provide space for detailed discussion, the present paper focuses on illustrative examples from two of a total of five aphasia assessment sessions, which were chosen as a way of demonstrating the full spectrum. One was conducted together with a Tagalog interpreter and involved the assessment of a trilingual Illocano-Tagalog-English speaker (approximately 80 years of age), while the second assessment involved a Vietnamese speaker (approximately 70 years of age) who also spoke some Cantonese. The time devoted to language assessment activities in these two encounters was 29 minutes and 40 minutes respectively.

Testing instrument

The testing instrument used in all assessments was the Western Aphasia Battery (Kertesz 1982) or WAB, reflecting the normal practice of speech pathologists at this particular institution when assessing aphasia. The WAB consists of two broad sections: (1) oral language subtests and (2) visual language and other subtests. The oral language subtests (some of which are being administered in the extracts considered in this paper) include spontaneous speech, auditory-verbal comprehension, repetition and naming.

Although the use of such aphasia test batteries with interpreters (who are asked to sight-translate the items) is sometimes criticized, it is the authors' experience that many speech pathologists opt to carry out an assessment which is parallel to that which they would conduct when assessing an English-speaking individual, which often means that a test such as the WAB is administered. The choice of assessment techniques and instruments in clinical situations such as these is a complex area, but one that falls outside the scope of the present paper (for a full discussion see Roger and Code 2011).

Data analysis

The recorded sessions were transcribed as far as possible by the first author, using the transcription conventions presented in the Appendix. The transcribed data was de-identified and pseudonyms were used for all participants. Where an understanding of the language of the assessment was necessary for this analysis, the assistance of bilingual speech pathologists was sought. As they were not professional interpreters, they were not asked to 'judge' the interpreters' performance or to back-translate every utterance, but instead to offer insights on what they saw in the sessions as speech pathologists who were able to access both languages directly. This could then be compared with information that the speech pathologist who carried out the assessment had received from the interpreter. Input from the bilingual speech pathologists proved extremely valuable, and is gratefully acknowledged. The transcripts were analysed for the following phenomena:

1. *Footing patterns*: positions that the speech pathologist or the interpreter adopt in the production or reception of an utterance (these

footing patterns in turn enabled the identification of three distinct frames – see below);

2. *Frame shifts*: points at which a change in the frame in operation at a particular time was triggered by one of the participants;
3. *Framing mismatches*: points at which the speech pathologist and the interpreter appeared to be operating in different frames, even for a single turn;
4. *Framing ambiguities*: places where the verbal or non-verbal behaviour of one or both professionals suggested that they were not sure which frame had been invoked by the other; and
5. *Different orientations within a frame*: where the interpreter and the speech pathologist appeared to agree on the general frame in operation at a given time, but did not seem to share a common understanding of the goals associated with that particular frame [= orientations] at that particular moment.

10.4 Findings

From the data analysed for this study, three key frames which characterize interpreter-mediated aphasia assessments were identified: the *Testing-Translating Frame*, the *Discussion-Description Frame* and the *Cultural-Linguistic Information Frame*. This was done by identifying the footings that the speech pathologist and the interpreter adopted towards each other in the reception and production formats.

The *Testing-Translating Frame* represents the 'default' frame for these encounters. The label reflects the normative roles of the two professionals: 'testing' (in the sense of language assessment) for the speech pathologist, and 'translation' for the interpreter. It is the default frame because within it both professionals are performing roles which are quite familiar to them (although they may or may not be used to working with each other). In terms of footing, the interpreter here tends to adopt a reporter's or recapitulator's footing in the reception format, thus producing utterances for which he or she is the animator or author (but not generally the principal).

The *Discussion-Description Frame* is invoked when the speech pathologist and/or interpreter find it necessary to engage in 'meta-talk' about what it is that they are doing. For example, it may be necessary for the interpreter to describe an aspect of an aphasic speaker's utterance that he or she has not been able to render into the language of the speech pathologist. Or, it may be necessary for a speech pathologist to instruct an interpreter (or seek his or her advice) on how a particular test item should be administered, or to seek extra information from the interpreter to assist with the assessment process. It thus involves a shift *away from* the usual testing role for the speech pathologist, and *away from* the semantic interpreting role for the interpreter. The interpreter here is addressed by the speech pathologist as a recapitulator or responder (rather than as a reporter), and thus responds not as an animator, but as an author or principal.

The *Cultural-Linguistic Information Frame* involves the professionals in sharing of information concerning linguistic features that cannot be tested in parallel across two or more languages; aphasia tests designed to test one language will inevitably run up against this barrier (to a greater or lesser extent) if they are translated/interpreted into other languages (Roger and Code 2011). Similarly, cultural differences can also make certain tests inappropriate or meaningless, even where a straight linguistic translation is possible. In this frame, the interpreter is ascribed the role of responder (in the reception format) and therefore assumes the role of principal in the production format.

These definitions are illustrated and substantiated in the extracts from the interactional discourse that follow. Our analysis of framing in the Tagalog encounter begins with an extract from the assessment session at a point where the speech pathologist is administering the repetition test from the WAB with the assistance of an interpreter (Extract 1). Because Pedro (the person with aphasia) understands and speaks English, hearing the test items in English before being asked to repeat the Tagalog translations (a procedure which is followed in some of the other assessments represented here, where the aphasic speaker has no knowledge of English) would complicate the test considerably, and make it difficult to interpret the results. Susan (the speech pathologist) thus 'hands over' the administration of the test to Iska (the interpreter), while she herself assumes a monitoring role. The initial items on the test are single words (e.g. banana, nose), and Extract 1 picks up the assessment as the items become longer and more complex.

Excerpt 1

1 Iska: *nobenta isinko porsiyento* [ninety-five percent]
2 Pedro: *nobenta isinko porsiyento* [ninety-five percent]
3 Iska: *sisentaidos at kalahate* [sixty-two and a half]

4	Pedro:	*sisentaidos e kalahate* [sixty-two and a half]
5	Susan:	((looks a little doubtful))
6	Iska:	*ang telepono ay tumutunog* [the telephone is ringing]
7	Pedro:	*ang telepono tumutunog* [the telephone ringing]
8	Susan:	that exactly the same?
9	Iska:	ah .. ringing … or .. sound .. making sound
10	Susan:	did ((inaudible)) change any words?
11	Iska:	no
12	Susan:	mm

At the item 'sixty-two and a half' Susan looks a little doubtful (turn 5) at the accuracy of Pedro's response, but does not interrupt at this stage. Analysis of the video recording does reveal a phonemic irregularity in Pedro's response; either this was not evident to Iska, or she did not think it worthy of comment, for she proceeded to the next item. Once again, there is some discrepancy between Iska's reading of the sentence and Pedro's repetition of it, and this time Susan chooses to stop the assessment to check with Iska on Pedro's performance, triggering a switch to the Discussion/Description Frame (turn 8).

It is at this point that the different expectations that each professional brings to the assessment become evident. Susan's question 'that exactly the same?' (turn 8) in the context of a repetition test almost certainly means 'did he repeat the sentence exactly as you said it?'. However, Iska (in her role as an interpreter) is oriented towards translating, not testing, so she takes the question as referring to the degree of equivalence achieved in her translation of 'ringing' as *tumutunog*. This can be clearly seen from her answer ('ah .. ringing … or .. sound .. making sound' – turn 9). Interestingly, Susan's follow-up question (with an unstressed pronoun – turn 10) sounds rather like 'did you change any words?' but is much more likely (in the context of a repetition test) to have been 'did he change any words?'. It is not clear what Iska's interpretation of this question is, but given her response to the previous question it seems likely that she has again taken it to refer to her translation, rather than to Pedro's performance. Thus, while Susan may have thought that the miscommunication had been repaired, some doubt remains as to whether this was in fact the case.

Once again, the expectations that arise from the different professionals' roles and knowledge schemata can be seen to influence the orientations of the participants when the Discussion/Description Frame is entered. Both seem to be aware that they are 'discussing and describing' but do not appear to be discussing or describing the same thing. The interpreter is oriented towards the translation issue of semantic equivalence (her own performance) while the speech pathologist is oriented toward the testing issue of repetition accuracy (the performance of the person with aphasia). It is for this reason that it becomes necessary to look *inside* the frame at the orientations of the two professionals in order to uncover the likely source of the misunderstanding.

As the repetition test progresses the items become longer, and the sentences move from being 'probable' (e.g. 'the telephone is ringing' – see Extract 1) to 'improbable' in Extract 2. Here, Iska hesitates when she encounters the test item 'the pastry cook was elated' and her hesitation prompts an exchange.

Excerpt 2

1	Susan:	just say 'happy' … happy's fine .. instead of 'elated' just say 'happy'
2	Iska:	*ang tagapagluto ay masaya* [the cook is happy]
3	Pedro:	*ang tag-pagluto masaya*
4	Susan:	clear?
5	Iska:	ah .. no .. not a bit .. not clear .. *tagapagluto* ((repeats more slowly in Tagalog for Pedro)) - *ang tagapagluto ay masaya*
6	Pedro:	*ang tagipagluto masaya*
7	Susan:	better that time .. or not?
8	Iska:	no .. no .. I mean, um … like .. it's a bit .. not .. ah .. there is like a ((inaudible))
9	Susan:	OK, this .. how does it sound different?
10	Iska:	no it's not different but ah .. you know it's just like ah .. like ..like stuttering … something like that
11	Susan:	⌊like stuttering on a sound
12	Iska:	yeah, yeah
13	Susan:	((writing)) - so it was happening at the beginning wasn't it
14	Iska:	yeah .. the cook .. I just said 'the cook'
15	Susan:	OK .. was it perhaps a bit fast, or ⌊something that … was making …
16	Iska:	⌊or maybe .. it's long ((inaudible)) =
17	Susan:	too long
18	Iska:	= long
19	Susan:	OK
20	Iska:	°I didn't get him to say the word 'pastry' anymore ((inaudible)) just .. the word 'cook'° =
21	Susan:	= cook .. yeah .. that's OK …

Susan triggers a frame shift with the question 'clear?' (turn 4). Iska replies that Pedro's repetition was not quite clear, and repeats the item to him again slowly. After he repeats it, Susan asks again about his performance (turn 7). Two points are notable with respect to Iska's contributions to the Discussion/Description Frame here.

The first point is the considerable difficulty that the focus on 'form' appears to pose for Iska. As was noted previously, interpreters would not normally be asked to attune their listening to focus on the formal features of a client's utterances in order to describe them. Thus when asked to do so, Iska can be seen to 'cast around' for words to describe what she has heard, before finally settling on the term 'stuttering'. This term has a specific technical meaning for speech pathologists, and the bilingual speech pathologist who assisted with the analysis was able to confirm that no stuttering was in fact apparent in this extract. The second point of interest is that, immediately following the discussion of the nature of Pedro's utterance, Iska reverts to the more familiar (for her) territory of semantic equivalence (turn 14, and again in turn 20). She stresses to Susan on both occasions that her translation of 'pastry cook' was semantically equivalent to the more general English term 'cook' (rather than 'pastry cook').

Extracts 3–5 come from an assessment of a Vietnamese woman with a severe fluent aphasia. The speech pathologist in this encounter is 'Simone', and the interpreter is 'Ian'. The person with aphasia is addressed with the title 'Mrs' plus surname by the speech pathologist, and is thus referred to here as 'Mrs Pham'. At the time of this assessment she had recently been discharged from hospital.

Extract 3 occurs several minutes into the assessment. The speech pathologist and the interpreter have already shifted on three occasions into the Discussion/Description Frame, and it has been established that much of Mrs Pham's speech consists of incomprehensible sounds with some discernable words interspersed. Ian's interpretation of Mrs Pham's utterance immediately preceding the extract below appears to contain well-expressed ideas (turn 2) and Simone thus asks (turn 3) the degree to which he had to 'work out' what she wanted to say.

Excerpt 3

1 Mrs Pham: *((fluent aphasic utterances))*
2 Ian: ((translating)) - oh right .. when I came home my grandchildren were very happy because, you know, they hadn't seen me for a long time ... so they gave me a big welcome
3 Simone: so was that something you had to try and work out or was that fairly clear then .. what she said

4 Ian: I don't know .. she just, you know, said something she want to talk
5 Simone: so when she just told you about her grandchildren, like, you understood clearly?
6 Ian: yep yep yep
7 Simone: it wasn't something you had to interpret or try and work out?
8 Ian: yep yep yep

At turn 4, Ian realizes that Simone has addressed him (in turn 3) as a responder, but it appears from his response that he believes that Simone is asking about the *topic* of Mrs Pham's utterance, when she is in fact asking Ian to reflect on how much work he had to do to guess and reconstruct her intended meaning. The two professionals appear to agree on the broad frame within which they are operating (labelled here the Discussion/Description Frame), but their orientations within this frame are clearly different.

The particular orientation adopted by the participants once again reflects the knowledge schemata associated with their respective professions. Being a non-Vietnamese speaker, Simone tries to gain an impression of how much work a native speaker must do to 'fill in the gaps' – as a speech pathologist, she is interested in the *form* of the aphasic speaker's utterances. In this case, the way in which an aphasic speaker's utterances strike their interlocutors is an important diagnostic factor in determining how 'functional' an individual's speech is. Ian, on the other hand, as an interpreter is normally oriented towards the *semantics* (*content*) of utterances. It appears that the meaning of Simone's question is initially unclear to him, and he thus resorts to reflection on the content rather than the form of Mrs Pham's speech.

Two other incidences of misunderstanding when moving out of the Testing/Translating Frame occur when the speech pathologist shifts frames to seek cultural or linguistic information from the interpreter (the Cultural/Linguistic Information Frame). In the first instance, shown in Extract 4, the speech pathologist interrupts her delivery of a test item (from the 'yes/no' question subtest) to check a detail (turn 1).

Excerpt 4

1 Simone: does it – ((softly to Ian)) - °in, in Vietnam does it snow in July?°
2 Ian: ((3 second pause)) °what do you mean?°
3 Simone: °does it snow in July in Vietnam?°
4 Ian: °no, no, never°
5 Simone: OK can you ask her ... in Vietnam does it snow in July?

The rapid frame shift appears to puzzle Ian here. Repeating the question and changing the order of the elements seems to clarify whatever was unclear; perhaps even a few seconds to think about the first question would have had the same effect. The second misunderstanding when moving into the Cultural/Linguistic Information Frame comes on the auditory word recognition subtest, where Mrs Pham is asked to point to various objects and body parts. Several items on this subtest have already been completed before the word 'thumb' comes up in Extract 5.

Excerpt 5

1	Simone:	thumb ... °say thumb?°
2	Ian:	[thumb]
3	Mrs Pham:	((wriggles fingers))
4	Simone:	do you have a differentiation?
5	Ian:	yeah?
6	Simone:	do you have a difference between thumb and fingers?
7	Ian:	no, no, no
8	Simone:	so she just showed me–
9	Ian:	no no no no this is **different** =
10	Simone	= there **is** a difference?
11	Ian:	different .. yeah ... different
12	Simone:	show me **just** your thumb

It is hard to speculate about Ian's reading of Simone's question in turn 4, as his first response is an ambiguous 'yeah?' with a rising intonation. Simone re-phrases the question, which he then answers emphatically with 'no no no'. Before Simone completes her follow-up checking question, Ian jumps in to clarify (turn 9), giving the impression that he has suddenly grasped the meaning of Simone's previous question.

Simone's use of 'you' (turn 4) may have contributed to the confusion here. In the Testing/Translating Frame, 'you' from the speech pathologist refers to the aphasic speaker. In the Discussion/Description Frame, 'you' from the speech pathologist refers to the interpreter. In the Cultural/Linguistic Information Frame, 'you' from the speech pathologist refers to 'Vietnamese speakers'. With such a rapid frame shift, it is possible that Ian mistook the re-framing to be a move to the Discussion/Description Frame, in which 'you' referred directly to him. This may have caused him to interpret words such as 'differentiation' and 'difference' as questions which related to his interpreting choices, rather than to possible differences between the English and Vietnamese languages. This would represent another instance of the interpreter taking a question to refer to his or her own performance in the 'normative' interpreting role, and a framing mismatch.

10.5 Discussion

The analysis presented above parallels the observations of Tannen and Wallat (1993) that mismatches in knowledge schemata constitute a force which tends to trigger frame shifts. Thus, for instance, the speech pathologist in the Vietnamese encounter initiated shifts into the Discussion/Description Frame because her lack of knowledge of the Vietnamese language meant that she could not distinguish 'unintelligible sounds' from speech which contained recognisable Vietnamese words or phrases. She also initiated shifts into the Cultural/Linguistic Information Frame when she needed to rely on the interpreter's knowledge of Vietnamese culture to determine the appropriateness of a particular test item. Similarly, the speech pathologist in the Tagalog encounter initiated frame shifts to check with the interpreter on the details of her client's production of Tagalog words and sentences on the repetition test.

Although the interpreters' responses on such occasions indicated that they tended to 'follow' the speech pathologist into the new frame, it was apparent that the two participants were at times differently oriented in their discussion. The most common pattern observed was one in which the speech pathologist's questions about the *form* of the speaker's utterances were answered by the interpreter with reference to the *semantic content* of these utterances, or the translation equivalents that they had chosen in the course of their own interpreting performance. This is directly traceable to the different knowledge schemata of the two professionals, as discussed at several points in this paper.

A very important point to recognize is that the competing demands of the Testing/Translating Frame (in which the interpreter must 'translate' test items and responses as well as keeping track of the structure of his or her own translations for the purpose of repetition) and the Discussion/Description Frame (where the interpreter is often asked to describe the *form* of disordered utterances) can place an excessive cognitive burden on the interpreter. This in turn can influence the orientation that the interpreter adopts (consciously or unconsciously), as the interpreter is forced by cognitive constraints to choose a focus. Because interpreters are uncertain at which points in the assessment they may suddenly be asked to respond to the speech pathologist as a principal (rather than an animator or author) in the production format, it is difficult for them to know exactly which mode of listening (reporter, recapitulator or responder) to adopt at various points during the encounter. The data presented here indicate that the outcome is frequently a situation in which the interpreter focuses on the aspects of language which are closest to his or her accustomed role (semantic meaning and equivalence) over those which are not (syntax and form). Hence, the interpreter's orientation may not match that of the speech pathologist. These professionals, like many interlocutors, are sensitive to cues that signal frame shifts, and it is only when one looks more deeply at the orientations inside the frame that reasons for the miscommunications become evident.

The present study has focused on discourse extracts which highlighted problematic aspects of the encounters, with a view to illuminating the roots of difficulties that both interpreters and speech pathologists frequently report when reflecting on such encounters. In doing so, however, it would be remiss not to mention the fact that the professionals involved in the encounters discussed here evidently put a great deal of effort into attempting to accommodate each other's needs. Furthermore, the willingness of the interpreters to work in a flexible mode and take on these complex interpreting/translation tasks for which they had little chance to prepare is admirable indeed, as without their assistance any assessment efforts would have been extremely limited. While the essence of the 'humane medical care' observed by Merlini and Favaron (2005) is also evident in the encounters recorded for the present study, the focus on problematic elements of the interactions will, it is hoped, provide practitioners the information that they need to come even closer to this ideal.

10.6 Conclusions and implications for practice

Speech pathologists who work with interpreters need to be aware that shifting frames to ask the interpreter for 'descriptions' of aphasic utterances can put the interpreter in a difficult position, for two reasons. First, it is likely that the interpreter has attended to the preceding utterance with the intention of rendering meaning into the language that the speech pathologist understands, and will therefore not have been attending to the precise details of the way in which the utterance was formed syntactically or phonologically. Secondly, such requests ask the interpreter to perform a task that extends (or even falls outside) their normal professional role. Speech pathologists should therefore forewarn interpreters that they may periodically seek such information, and explain why this is necessary. Interpreters too should share with the speech pathologist information of a cultural or linguistic nature that they feel is relevant, and raise with the speech pathologist any concerns or points that they would like clarified. A pre-session briefing is the ideal forum for working through these issues, and (as Isaac 2002 points out) such briefings should allow for the active participation of both parties so that they are genuinely collaborative in nature.

Based on the analysis presented above, it is argued that a more fundamental re-organization of the interpreter-mediated aphasia assessment would enhance the quality of information to emerge from the assessment, while reducing both the cognitive burden on the interpreter and the need for the person with aphasia to be sidelined frequently during the assessment. This re-working would involve two sessions: at the first session, the speech pathologist and the interpreter would engage in a pre-session briefing; this would be followed by a clinical encounter with the person with aphasia during which the chosen aphasia tests would be administered with minimal requests for description by the speech pathologist. The session would be video-recorded, so that the speech pathologist and interpreter could (at a second session) watch the video together and engage in extensive discussion and description. The interpreter would therefore be able to adopt the more usual footing of recapitulator/reporter during the initial session, without the pressure of being suddenly called upon to 'respond' as a principal without warning. Frequent frame shifts in which the individual with aphasia were put 'on hold' would also be avoided. At the second session (involving only the speech pathologist and interpreter), crucial segments of the recording could be re-played as many times as necessary for the interpreter and the speech pathologist to hone in on specific features that may be impossible for the interpreter to monitor while carrying out the task of interpreting.

This sort of re-organization would obviously require the sanction of the individual interpreters concerned, which would also have both time and financial implications for the professionals and the healthcare system. To ensure true equity of access to speech pathology services in situations where interpreting is necessary, however, it is vital that novel approaches are considered so that the loss of valuable diagnostic information is minimized.

Appendix: Transcription conventions

..	two dots indicate a short pause (< 1 second)
...	three dots indicate a longer pause (> 1 second)
telepono	italics indicate a language other than English
[banana]	square brackets indicate a back-translation into English
((laughs))	double parentheses indicate a non-verbal cue or transcriber's comment
have	bold type indicates a word spoken with emphasis
⌈or ⌊right	latches indicate overlapping speech
=	an equal sign indicates an interruption
,	a comma indicates that the intonation suggests that the speaker will continue
li–	a long dash indicates an incomplete word

References

Beck, Christina S. and Sandra L. Ragan (1992) Negotiating interpersonal and medical talk: Frame shifts in the gynaecologic exam. *Journal of Language and Social Psychology* 11 (1–2): 47–61. https://doi.org/10.1177/0261927X92111004

Clark, Elizabeth (1998) *Interpreting for Speech Pathology: An Ethnographic Study.* Unpublished Master's dissertation, University of Melbourne, Melbourne, Australia.

Coupland, Nikolas and Adam Jaworski (1997) Relevance, accommodation and conversation: Modeling the social dimension of communication. *Multilingua* 16 (2–3): 233–258. https://doi.org/10.1515/mult.1997.16.2-3.233

Coupland, Justine, Jeffrey D. Robinson and Nikolas Coupland (1994) Frame negotiation in doctor-elderly patient consultations. *Discourse and Society* 5 (1): 89–124. https://doi.org/10.1177/0957926594005001005

Frey, Roger, Len Roberts-Smith and Susan Bessell-Browne (1990) *Working with Interpreters in Law, Health and Social Work.* Canberra: National Accreditation Authority for Translators and Interpreters.

Gentile, Adolfo, Uldis Ozolins and Mary Vasilakakos (1996) *Liaison Interpreting.* Melbourne: Melbourne University Press.

Goffman, Erving (1974) *Frame Analysis: An Essay on the Organization of Experience.* New York: Harper & Row.

Goodglass, Harold and Edith Kaplan (1983) *Boston Diagnostic Aphasia Examination* (2nd edition). Philadelphia: Lea and Febiger.

Goodwin, Charles (1981) *Conversational Organization: Interaction between Speakers and Hearers.* New York: Academic Press.

Goodwin, Charles (2000) Action and embodiment within situated human interaction. *Journal of Pragmatics* 32 (10): 1499–1522. https://doi.org/10.1016/S0378-2166(99)00096-X

Halvorsen, Kristin and Srikant Sarangi (2015) Team decision-making in workplace meetings: The interplay of activity roles and discourse roles. *Journal of Pragmatics* 76: 1–14. https://doi.org/10.1016/j.pragma.2014.11.002

Isaac, Kim (2002) *Speech Pathology in Cultural and Linguistic Diversity.* London: Whurr Publications.

Kertesz, Andrew (1982) *The Western Aphasia Battery.* New York: Grune and Stratton.

Merlini, Raffaela and Roberta Favaron (2005) Examining the 'Voice of Interpreting' in speech pathology. *Interpreting* 7 (2): 263–302. https://doi.org/10.1075/intp.7.2.07mer

National Accreditation Authority for Translators and Interpreters (2000) *Ethics of Translation and Interpreting: A Guide to Professional Conduct in Australia.* Canberra: NAATI.

Ribeiro, Branca Telles (1993) Framing in psychotic discourse. In Deborah Tannen (ed.) *Framing in Discourse*, 77–113. New York: Oxford University Press.

Ribeiro, Branca T. and Liliana C. Bastos (2005) Telling stories in two psychiatric interviews: A discussion on frame and narrative. *AILA Review* 18 (1): 58–75. https://doi.org/10.1075/aila.18.06tel

Roger, Peter and Chris Code (2011) Lost in translation? Issues of content validity in interpreter-mediated aphasia assessments. *International Journal of Speech-Language Pathology* 13 (1): 61–73. https://doi.org/10.3109/17549507.2011.549241

Roger, Peter, Chris Code and Christine Sheard (2000) Assessment and management of aphasia in a linguistically diverse society. *Asia Pacific Journal of Speech, Language and Hearing* 5 (1): 21–34. https://doi.org/10.1179/136132800807547573

Sarangi, Srikant (2015) Experts on experts: Sustaining 'communities of interest' in professional discourse studies. In Maurizio Gotti, Stefania M. Maci and Michele Sala (eds) *Insights into Medical Communication*, 25–47. Bern: Peter Lang.

Siyambalapitiya, Samantha and Bronwyn Davidson (2015) Managing aphasia in bilingual and culturally and linguistically diverse individuals in an

Australian context. *Journal of Clinical Practice in Speech-Language Pathology* 17 (1): 13–19.

Speech Pathology Australia (n.d.) *Fact Sheet: How do Speech Pathologists work in a Multilingual and Culturally Diverse Society?* Available online: http://www.speechpathologyaustralia.org.au/library/4.1_How_do_Speech_Pathologists_work_in_a_Multilingual_Culturally_Diverse_Society.pdf

Tannen, Deborah and Cynthia Wallat (1993) Interactive frames and knowledge schemas in interaction: Examples from a medical examination/interview. In Deborah Tannen (ed.) *Framing in Discourse*, 57–76. New York: Oxford University Press.

Thomassen, Goril (2009) The role of role-play: Managing activity ambiguities in simulated doctor consultation in medical education. *Communication & Medicine* 6 (1): 83–93. https://doi.org/10.1558/cam.v6i1.83

Wadensjö, Cecelia (1998) *Interpreting as Interaction*. Harlow, UK: Addison Wesley Longman.

Whitworth, Anne and Helen Sjardin (1993) The bilingual person with aphasia – The Australian context. In Denise Lafond, Yves Joanette, Jacques Ponzio, René DeGiovani and Martha Taylor Sarno (eds) *Living with Aphasia: Psychosocial Issues*, 129–150. San Diego, CA: Singular Publishing Group.

Peter Roger is an Associate Professor in Linguistics at Macquarie University. A medical graduate from the University of Sydney, he worked as a medical practitioner for several years before going on to complete a PhD in communication sciences and disorders. His research interests include communication in healthcare contexts, and individual differences in second language acquisition. He is co-author (with Sally Candlin) of *Communication and Professional Relationships in Healthcare Practice* (Equinox, 2013). Address for correspondence: Department of Linguistics, Macquarie University, NSW, Australia 2109. E-mail: peter.roger@mq.edu.au

Chris Code is Professorial Research Fellow in the Department of Psychology, University of Exeter and Foundation Professor of Communication Sciences and Disorders at the University of Sydney (1992–1998). He is the co-founding editor of the international journal *Aphasiology*. His research interests include the cognitive neuroscience of language and speech, psychosocial consequences of aphasia, aphasia and the evolution of language and speech, recovery and treatment of aphasia and public awareness of aphasia. Address for correspondence: Department of Psychology, Washington Singer Laboratories, University of Exeter, Perry Road, Exeter, EX4 4QG, UK.
E-mail: c.f.s.code@exeter.ac.uk

Author Index

Subject Index